THE HARVARD UNIVERSITY PRESS FAMILY HEALTH GUIDES

# Parkinson's Disease and the Family

## A NEW GUIDE

Nutan Sharma, M.D.
Elaine Richman, Ph.D.

HARVARD UNIVERSITY PRESS
Cambridge, Massachusetts
London, England
2005

Illustrations by Arleen Frasca

Cataloging-in-Publication Data available from the Library of Congress

Sharma, Nutan.
   Parkinson's disease and the family : a new guide / Nutan Sharma, Elaine
Richman.
      p.   cm.—(The Harvard University Press family health guides)
   Includes bibliographical references and index.
   ISBN 0-674-01679-3 (cloth : alk. paper)—ISBN 0-674-01751-X (paper : alk.
paper)
   1. Parkinson's disease—Popular works.   I. Richman, Elaine.   II. Title.
III. Series.
RC382.S48  2005
616.8′33—dc22        2005040346

Nutan Sharma dedicates this book to her parents, Moti Lal and
Krishan Kanta Sharma, whose unstinting support gave her the
opportunity to become a neurologist, and to her husband, Antonio J.
Aldykiewicz, Jr., and her son, Vikram E. Aldykiewicz, whose unstinting support allows her to continue her work as a neurologist.

Elaine Richman dedicates this book to her good friend Dr. Charles P.
Barrett, whose Parkinson's disease helped her understand the condition, and to her loving husband, Ralph Raphael, and children, David
and Matt Richman-Raphael.

# Contents

PARKINSON'S DISEASE AND THE FAMILY

# Introduction

*Ken was embarrassed by his father's funny gait and slow way of talk-ing. His dad, though, had a way of making everyone think that he was managing just fine.*

*Marissa was one of the first people Sue told about her husband's diagnosis of Parkinson's disease. What Sue wanted most was the unconditional support of a friend with whom she could share her worries.*

Parkinson's disease (PD) is a chronic and progressive condi-tion that affects not only the person with the disease but also his or her loved ones. Everyone reacts differently to a diagnosis of PD—the person with the condition, the spouse, partner, chil-dren, extended family, coworkers, and friends. No one can tell you how to feel or how to behave, but as you talk with more and more people about Parkinson's disease, you will find common threads in everyone's experience.

We recommend that you embark on your journey with Par-kinson's disease by gathering information. Start with the ba-sics: anatomy, symptoms, course of the disease, psychological aspects, and so on. There will be a lot of decisions ahead, and they are best made when you know the facts. Families say that a search for facts gives them comfort and a sense of control. If you are new to Parkinson's disease, you will soon see that you have joined a large community of passionately supportive health care providers, researchers, families, and advocacy groups.

Modern medicine has made tremendous strides in the last century, contributing to our increased lifespan and an improved quality of life for those with chronic illnesses. Our knowledge of the human body and how it malfunctions has grown exponentially. The result is that highly skilled, knowledgeable, and compassionate care is available from highly trained medical professionals. The difficulty, however, is in how to convey this knowledge and the wide array of potential treatments to people affected by the disease.

The goal of this book is to provide straightforward information to the general public about what is known about Parkinson's disease and its treatment. This book is meant for people with Parkinson's disease and their friends and family members. We do not live in isolation, despite the ubiquity of television and the Internet, and it is important for everyone involved in the life of someone with Parkinson's disease to understand the illness. Fortunately, we no longer live in a society where people are afraid to discuss disease. Knowledge is essential to minimize fear. We hope that the information in this book will help make people less fearful about Parkinson's disease and more likely to become actively involved in their own treatment or that of a loved one.

The first several chapters contain medical information, in plain English, that describes what we know about the causes of Parkinson's disease and the many aspects of its treatment. They also contain practical information that should help answer some of the most common questions that arise about daily life: questions about driving, travel, work, intimacy, mental health, alternative medicine, and so on. The patient anecdotes that are found throughout the book illustrate the problems faced by many families coping with the diagnosis of Parkinson's disease.

As a movement disorder neurologist, I (Dr. Sharma) have had

the pleasure of developing long-term relationships with many patients and the people closest to them. It is a great joy to hear news of family weddings, the birth of grandchildren, and other special life events. People with PD generally live with the disease for many years, and so I have met and spoken at length with many family members and friends of my patients. I count among the greatest privileges in the practice of medicine the opportunity to work with whole families, to coach them in coping with illness, and to help them live as active and independent lives as possible.

Throughout this book, we have tried to address the concerns of friends and family members as well as those with Parkinson's disease. We have tried to shed light on what the diagnosis means to everyone within the family unit and explore what the responses and fears of others may be. It is our hope that this book will serve as a springboard for family talks and for open and meaningful discussions between patients and physicians.

# 1

# What Is Parkinson's Disease?

Parkinson's disease has troubled people since ancient times. Early books from China and India describe patients whose symptoms we recognize. The first modern description of PD appeared in 1817 in a paper by a London physician named James Parkinson. He called the paper "An Essay on the Shaking Palsy." He summarized what he saw in this way:

> The patient can [rarely] form any recollection of the precise period of its commencement. The first symptoms perceived are, a slight sense of weakness, with a proneness to trembling in some particular part; sometimes in the head, but most commonly in one of the hands and arms . . . The propensity to lean forward becomes invincible . . . As the debility increases and the influence of the will over the muscles fades away, the tremulous agitation becomes more vehement.

When most of us think of Parkinson's disease, we think of the uncontrollable shaking of an arm or a leg. This is true, and it is much more.

The shaking, or tremor, is one of the four cardinal signs of Parkinson's disease. The term *cardinal sign* refers to the physical features that are seen in the vast majority of men and women with PD. Parkinson's disease affects people from every nation of the world. In the United States alone, more than 1.2 million people have Parkinson's disease and nearly 50,000 new cases are diagnosed each year.

Parkinson's disease is one of the most common neurological ailments in North America. One of the predominant factors contributing to this phenomenon is that people are living longer. (Our average life span has increased from 50 years in 1900 to an all-time high of 77.2 years in 2001.)[1] Because Parkinson's disease is typically an illness of the middle and later years, it is not surprising that the number of older people with Parkinson's disease is increasing. The "baby boomers" are growing older. As the proportion of Americans over the age of 55 grows, so will the number of Americans with Parkinson's disease.

Parkinson's disease belongs to a class of diseases called movement disorders. A movement disorder is a neurological condition in which a person gradually loses control of voluntary movements like walking or sitting quietly or using a pen. (See Figure 1.)

Scientists and physicians describe two basic categories of movement disorders. One is characterized by unusual or excess activity. The other is characterized by slowness or absence of movement. Parkinson's disease fits into the second category because people with the condition often move slowly and deliberately. The terms *hypokinesia, bradykinesia,* and *akinesia* are sometimes used to refer to a condition such as Parkinson's disease where movement is slow or absent.

Parkinson's disease is a chronic and progressive condition. This means that it persists for a long period and that the symptoms grow progressively worse. It is not contagious; nor is it inherited, except in a very small number of cases. In the vast majority of cases, PD is not passed on from parent to child, so worrying about heredity is unwarranted. Although there are a

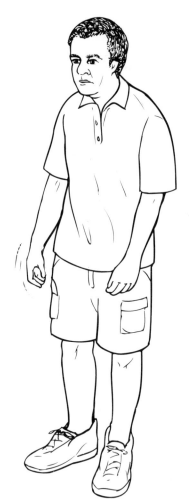

FIGURE 1.   A person with Parkinson's disease. Note the slightly stooped posture and tremor involving one arm.

set of symptoms that affect people with Parkinson's disease, it is important to realize that not everyone is impacted in the same way or to the same extent.

There are no laboratory tests for diagnosing Parkinson's disease. A physician usually examines a patient several times over a period of twelve to twenty-four months before making the diagnosis, to be sure that the symptoms do not belong to one of several other diseases that resemble PD.

In some people, Parkinson's disease develops slowly. In others, the progression of symptoms is rapid. Symptoms may be minor or disabling. Each patient's experience is unique. In the sections that follow we provide information to help all patients and their families cope with the inevitable changes they experience after a diagnosis of PD.

## The Anatomy of Parkinson's Disease

Parkinson's disease is a neurological condition resulting from the death of cells in a portion of the brain called the basal ganglia. In the early 1960s scientists conclusively linked the loss of brain cells of the basal ganglia to symptoms of Parkinson's disease. (See Figure 2a–2c.)

Every portion of the brain plays a unique role. The basal ganglia is responsible for maintaining body posture, muscle tone, and smooth, purposeful muscle activity—movements we normally perform without even thinking, such as walking. An abnormality in the basal ganglia results in poorly regulated muscle movements and other signs that we will discuss later.

Specific cells within the basal ganglia normally produce dopamine, a chemical messenger that is responsible for transmitting signals to other portions of the brain. In people with Parkinson's disease these dopamine-producing cells die off. The cornerstone of treatment for PD is the replacement of dopamine, the chemical messenger that is no longer produced because the cells responsible for its production have died. (See Figure 3.)

When dopamine is low, nerve cells of the basal ganglia transmit signals abnormally, making it difficult for a person to control muscle movements. The cause of the nerve cell death is

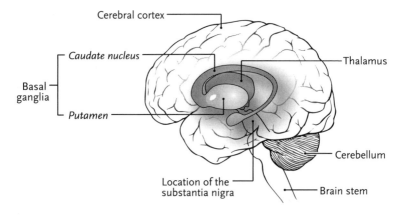

FIGURE 2A.    Profile of the brain. The *cerebral cortex* consists of the cells on the surface of the brain. These cells are involved in the ability to think, remember, learn new things, understand language, and express oneself. The *thalamus* is often referred to as the "Grand Central Station" of the brain. This is where information from nerve cells throughout the body comes in, gets organized, and then routes to different regions of the brain. The *cerebellum* is the area that controls coordination, such as the ability to walk a straight line or reach out with two fingers and pick one flower out of an arrangement. The *brain stem* is the area that controls the most basic, vital functions, such as breathing, heart rate, and blood pressure. The *basal ganglia* is a collection of brain cells that control and modify movement. Some components of the basal ganglia include the *caudate nucleus,* the *putamen,* and the *substantia nigra.* In Parkinson's disease, dopamine-producing cells of the substantia nigra degenerate.

not known, but scientists are studying several theories. One theory relates to free radicals; another concerns environmental toxins. Also under investigation are genetic factors and the possibility of a premature aging of the dopamine-producing brain cells.

Free radicals are molecules formed by the body as it goes

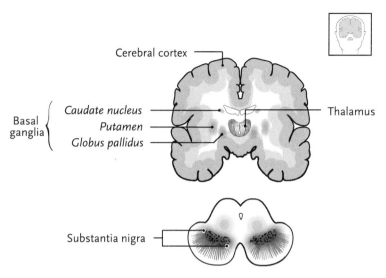

Cerebral cortex

Basal ganglia
Caudate nucleus
Putamen
Globus pallidus

Thalamus

Substantia nigra

FIGURE 2B.    Cross-section of the brain. In the upper panel is an additional component of the basal ganglia, the *globus pallidus*. Each component of the basal ganglia contains many brain cells that communicate with cells in other regions of the basal ganglia. In the lower panel is a cross-section of the portion of the brain containing the substantia nigra. Cells in the substantia nigra produce dopamine and melanin; the melanin is responsible for the dark color of this region.

about its constant task of breaking down food, repairing injuries, maintaining normal metabolism, and so forth. Free radicals are highly reactive and, as such, have the potential to cause damage. Every cell in the body can cope with and repair a small amount of damage caused by free radicals. Fortunately, most free radical molecules are "mopped up" by being bound to other molecules, termed "antioxidants," which serve to stabilize and thus inactivate the free radical. If free radicals are not able to bind to substances such as iron to become stable, they go on to interact with and damage other molecules within a cell. The pro-

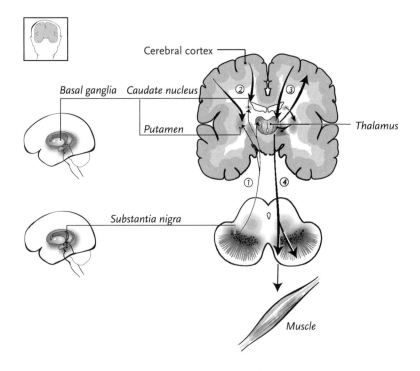

FIGURE 2C.   Connections between various brain regions and how they control movement. Consider what is involved in lifting your right thumb. (1) Information from the substantia nigra goes to the putamen, thalamus, and caudate nucleus. (2) The instruction "lift the right thumb" goes from the cerebral cortex to the putamen and caudate nucleus. (3) Information is exchanged between the thalamus, caudate, globus pallidus, putamen, and cortex, to determine how far to lift the right thumb (quarter-inch or half-inch) and at what angle (30 degrees or 45 degrees). (4) The final instruction, to lift the right thumb by a quarter-inch at a 45 degree angle, is then sent out to the body.

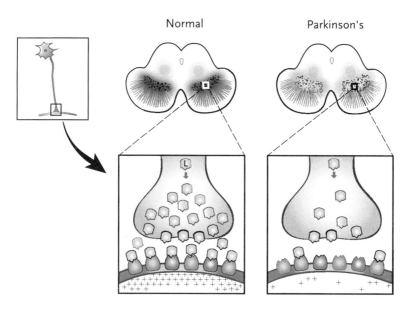

Normal                          Parkinson's

FIGURE 3.    The substantia nigra in a healthy individual and in someone with Parkinson's disease. The left panel depicts a normal substantia nigra. The brain section is dark because the cells are healthy
and produce both melanin and dopamine. A detailed diagram of the
nerve ending depicts dopamine being released from one cell and then
binding to its specific receptors on the adjacent cell.

   The right panel depicts the substantia nigra in an individual with
Parkinson's disease. The brain section is pale because the cells producing melanin and dopamine have died off. At the nerve ending,
only small amounts of dopamine are being made and released.

cess in which free radicals damage other molecules in a cell is
called oxidation. If the oxidation process continues unchecked,
cells that are not able to stabilize the free radical molecules can
die. The death of cells in the substantia nigra as a result of excessive oxidation is thought to play a role in the development of Parkinson's disease. One possible way to limit the damage caused

by oxidation is to eat a diet rich in antioxidants or to take antioxidant vitamin supplements. Several antioxidant compounds have been or are in the process of being studied as potential treatments for PD. This will be discussed further in Chapter 11.

Attention to environmental toxins as a cause of Parkinson's disease gained steam in the 1980s when several people who used illicit drugs developed Parkinson's-like paralysis after injecting themselves with a synthetic narcotic. Scientists found that the substance was MPTP (1-methyl-4-phenyl-1,2,3,6-tetra-hydropyridine), a toxin that accumulates inside dopamine nerve cells at a very high level and destroys the cells by interfering with the functioning of mitochondria, the "batteries" within each of our cells that produce the energy that cells need to survive. MPTP acts as a poison in the mitochondria, resulting in decreased energy production and cell death. Because the chemical structure of MPTP is similar to that of dopamine, MPTP is taken up and concentrated in dopamine-producing neurons within the brain. This results in the death of those neurons while the rest of the brain cells, and most of the cells throughout the body, continue to function.

Another theory examines genetic factors in causing a form of Parkinson's disease that occurs typically but not always in people under 40. Some people in this group have a close relative who exhibits Parkinson-like symptoms such as tremors.

Scientists are also looking at the possibility that the dopamine-producing brain cells in people with Parkinson's disease age faster than normal. This theory is supported by the fact that the loss of antioxidant protective mechanisms is associated with both aging and Parkinson's disease.

Perhaps scientists will discover that some or all of these events contribute to the development of Parkinson's disease. Researchers are aggressively exploring causes and possible treatments for PD. The National Institutes of Health support a variety of research programs directed toward both understanding the cause and finding new treatments.

## Signs and Symptoms of Parkinson's Disease

A *sign* of a disease is that which is evident to a physician during a physical examination. For example, bradykinesia, or slowness of movement, can be a sign of Parkinson's disease. A *symptom* of a disease is a subjective experience described by the patient that is not evident to an outside observer. For example, an aching muscle can be a symptom of Parkinson's disease. (See Table 1.)

People with Parkinson's disease typically first notice changes in the way they walk or feel. They usually wait a while before bringing the problem to the attention of their physician.

When people finally put words to the symptoms, they might talk about feeling shaky and clumsy, sore, and tired or depressed. Parkinson's disease can be confused with a number of other conditions, so the doctor will be looking for the cardinal signs of the disorder. As mentioned above, physicians use the term *cardinal signs* to describe features that are most common in people with a given disease. In Parkinson's disease, these signs

*Table 1*   Motor and nonmotor signs and symptoms of Parkinson's disease

| Motor | Nonmotor |
| --- | --- |
| Bradykinesia | Anxiety |
| Dystonia | Cognitive abnormalities |
| Gait difficulty | Depression |
| Rest tremor | Hallucinations, delusions, psychosis |
| Rigidity | Sexual dysfunction |
| | Sleep disturbances |
| | Urinary incontinence |

are all caused by the loss of cells that produce dopamine in the basal ganglia of the brain.

There are four cardinal signs of Parkinson's disease:

- rest tremor
- rigidity
- bradykinesia
- changes in posture and gait

### Rest Tremor

A tremor is a rhythmic and involuntary shaking of a part of the body. There are many different kinds of tremors, the most common of which is called an essential tremor (ET). An essential tremor occurs mostly in the hands, forearms, and head, when that part of the body is in motion or held in a specific position. The legs and torso are rarely involved. Essential tremor is often confused with the tremor of Parkinson's disease. The tremor of PD is called a rest tremor because it occurs when the affected body part is at rest and the muscles are relaxed. It is important to distinguish between different types of tremors so that a doctor can prescribe the most effective treatment.

A thorough neurological exam can usually distinguish between a Parkinson rest tremor and the less serious ET. ET is diagnosed in people who show a visible and persistent tremor that occurs when their arms or head are in a specific position or when they move. An essential tremor is *not* present when the arms are at rest. Although ET tends to worsen with age, it is *not* associated with the other neurological symptoms that occur with Parkinson's disease, like bradykinesia and loss of postural reflexes. Most cases of essential tremor are hereditary. The rest tremor of Parkinson's disease typically begins in a hand or foot and is intermittent. You may have heard the tremor described as a "pill-rolling" action because of the characteristic rolling movement of the thumb and opposing fingers.

Over time, the rest tremor spreads until all four limbs are involved. Because the rest tremor disappears or decreases during movement, it does not interfere with the ability to perform everyday tasks like walking or grasping objects. It is present in 70 to 80 percent of people with Parkinson's disease and may also appear in the face and jaw. A rest tremor is often more pronounced on one side of the body than the other. It typically responds well to medication.

### Rigidity

Rigidity refers to stiffness that occurs in the arms or legs. It is not unusual for people with Parkinson's disease to first complain of soreness in an arm or leg, which they usually attribute to muscle strain. As the sensations of soreness and stiffness persist, it becomes clear that a more pervasive disorder is the underlying cause.

Rigidity develops when the natural contraction and relaxation of opposing muscles fails to take place. Every muscle has a nearby muscle that opposes it; normally, when one muscle contracts, its opposite muscle relaxes. Rigidity occurs when this balance is disturbed.

### Bradykinesia

Bradykinesia means slowness of movement. In general, a person with PD will complain of slowness in performing routine activities like dressing, eating, and walking. Many people with Parkinson's disease never experience a rest tremor but do experience marked bradykinesia and rigidity. In addition to a loss of speed in Parkinson's disease, there is also a decline in the amplitude of repeated movements; that is, for example, a person with Parkinson's disease takes smaller and smaller steps the farther he or she walks.

### Posture and Gait

Loss of postural reflexes is the fourth cardinal sign of Parkinson's disease. This condition causes problems with balance. In particular, people with Parkinson's disease have a tendency to fall backward, usually because they do not lean far enough forward as they stand up. Thus their center of gravity falls behind where their feet are, resulting in the tendency to lean backward and fall.

## As if That Were Not Enough

A number of secondary signs and symptoms can occur in people with Parkinson's disease. As we stated above, not everyone with Parkinson's disease develops the same symptoms. Each of these secondary signs and symptoms will be discussed in detail in later chapters of this book:

- *Masked facies.* Some people with Parkinson's disease may experience a loss of facial expression and a decreased rate of eye blinking. (See Figure 4.)
- *Dysarthric speech.* Speech may become slow, slurred, soft, and monotonous.
- *Micrographia.* Handwriting may become small because of difficulty with fine motor movement.
- *Dysphagia.* Parkinson's disease can affect the muscles involved in swallowing. A common problem early in the course of Parkinson's disease is mild difficulty swallowing, with the food staying in the mouth for a longer period than

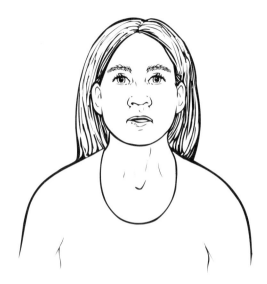

FIGURE 4.    The masked facies of PD. Note the abscence of wrinkles on the forehead, the wide-open stare, and the lack of facial expression.

usual. In those whose Parkinson's disease has progressed, the muscles do not work in a coordinated fashion and food may end up "going down the wrong pipe" into the airway and lungs rather than into the esophagus and stomach.

- *Drooling.* Healthy individuals swallow unconsciously throughout the day, which allows the saliva in their mouths to enter the stomach. Because people with PD have difficulty swallowing, saliva tends to build up in their mouths and can result in drooling.
- *Gastrointestinal complications.* Most people with Parkinson's disease experience constipation.
- *Skin problems.* Increased sweating may occur and skin may become oily.
- *Mental health.* Depression is the most common psychological problem in Parkinson's disease. It affects about 40 per-

cent of people with PD. Anxiety and cognitive disorders such as memory loss may also occur.

There is no doubt that Parkinson's disease is an enormous challenge. By reading this first chapter, you have taken an important and positive step toward meeting it.

# 2

# The Diagnosis

*Mr. Chaban is a seventy-four-year-old man who comes to the doctor's office with his adult son, Jonathan. Mr. Chaban is a widower who recently sold his home and moved in with Jonathan, his daughter-in-law, and two grandchildren.*

*Mr. Chaban says that after his children grew and moved out he and his wife had coped "just fine." However, more detailed questioning reveals that Mr. Chaban stopped driving two years ago. At about the same time, his wife started to take care of the bills because Mr. Chaban's handwriting had become illegible. After his wife died, Mr. Chaban moved in with his son because he felt "weak" all the time and was uncomfortable going up and down the stairs when he was alone in his own house.*

*Jonathan noticed that Mr. Chaban was taking an hour each morning to shower, shave, and dress. At the dinner table, Mr. Chaban would ask for his daughter-in-law's help in cutting food (a sign of decreased fine-motor dexterity). Jonathan also noticed that the booming voice he remembered from his father's younger days had become soft and difficult to understand. The symptoms that Jonathan described are confirmed on examination by a neurologist, who detects bradykinesia (slowness of movement), micrographia (decreased size of letters when writing), and hypophonia (soft voice).*

The diagnosis of Parkinson's disease is based on a physical exam completed by an experienced doctor, often a neurologist who specializes in movement disorders. The most common initial signs of Parkinson's disease are rest tremor and/or bradykinesia. Less common symptoms are also possible, like hypophonia, gait problems, and fatigue. It is typical for one of these symptoms to be present for months or even years before others develop.

Physicians use standard scales for rating a person's disability from Parkinson's disease. The most common scales are used worldwide for evaluating the disease symptoms and a patient's ability to manage independently. The Hoehn and Yahr Scale, the Unified Parkinson's Disease Rating Scale, and the Schwab and England Activities of Daily Living Scale are described in detail later in the chapter.

Keep in mind that Parkinson's disease is a disorder that develops slowly. It is estimated that 60 percent of dopamine-producing neurons are lost before the onset of symptoms. Once symptoms develop, the course of the disease varies remarkably from one person to another. So what does this mean if you or someone you love has Parkinson's disease? It means that from one doctor's visit to another you should not compare scores on any given rating scale. For example, if the score worsens by five points in one year, that does not mean that the score will continue to worsen by 5 points or more in subsequent years. Disease progression is unpredictable. Some people have spent more than ten years with minimal disease or more than twenty years with only slightly more severe symptoms.

## Rest Tremor

To evaluate a rest tremor, a physician may use one of several techniques. To observe a hand tremor, the doctor might ask a patient to walk with hands relaxed along the side of the body, or to lie on an exam table, where the hand tremor will often become more obvious. To elicit a leg tremor, the doctor may ask a seated patient to cross his or her legs. This typically unmasks a rest tremor involving the upper leg.

A doctor will also want to review medical history, medication history, and possible exposure to toxic compounds because some diseases, medications, and poisons can also cause tremor. Hyperthyroidism, a medical condition in which the thyroid gland is overactive, is an example of an underlying illness that can cause tremor. The following drugs and toxins can also cause tremor:

- alcohol
- antipsychotics such as haloperidol (Haldol), chlorpromazine (Thorazine), and olanzapine (Zyprexa)
- caffeine
- lithium
- nicotine
- valproate sodium (Depakene, Depacon)

Some of these agents will cause shaking that very closely resembles a Parkinson rest tremor.

## Bradykinesia

Bradykinesia can be tested by asking a person to open and close the fist, say ten times. Try it and you will see that normally, if you do not have Parkinson's disease, your hand will open completely. Fingers spread and extend, and each time your hand opens to the same extent that it did the time before. In someone with Parkinson's disease, initially the fingers may be spread and open but, with each subsequent try, the range of movement is diminished. Instead of extending, the fingers bend; instead of spreading apart, they nearly meet. Many patients with Parkinson's disease do not even realize that their movements are incomplete. Decreased swinging of the arms during walking and a shuffling gait are related phenomena.

Slow movement is not unique to Parkinson's disease. Several other conditions can cause bradykinesia, and a doctor will want to rule them out. Here are other possible causes of slow movement:

- arthritis
- "boxers' encephalopathy," caused by repeated head trauma
- cerebrovascular disease
- dementia
- depression

The slowness of Parkinson's disease is typically asymmetric, that is, one side of the body is more affected than the other. This may be obvious to the patient and family, but the doctor will want to confirm it by having the patient open and close both the right and the left fists.

## Gait Difficulty

The gait associated with Parkinson's disease typically consists of short, shuffling steps in which the heel is not put down completely on the floor. In addition, the head and shoulders are stooped, causing an individual to look down rather than forward. The arms also tend to stay rigidly at one's side rather than swinging in cadence with the legs. (See Figure 5.)

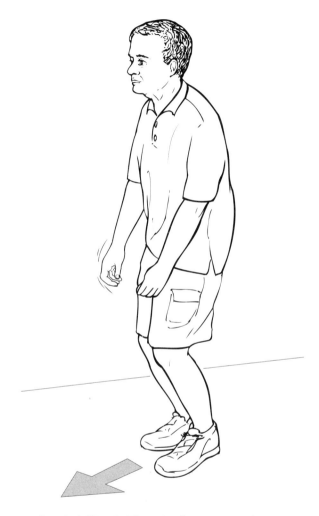

FIGURE 5.    A typical PD gait. The gait of someone with PD is generally characterized by stooped shoulders, an arm tremor or minimal movement of the arm on the affected side, and small, shuffling steps.

## Dystonia

Dystonia refers to the uncontrolled contraction of counteracting muscles in a particular part of the body. The most common form of dystonia in people with Parkinson's disease is seen as their medications wear off. Foot cramping is a common dystonic problem that is caused by uncontrolled contraction of muscles of the toes and sole of the foot.

*Elena was a sixty-two-year-old woman who had been diagnosed with Parkinson's disease six years earlier. At that time, she noticed some stiffness and slowness mostly in her right arm and right leg. As an elementary school teacher, Elena wrote on the board frequently throughout the day. Her students and aide began to complain that her handwriting was becoming difficult to read. She was diagnosed with Parkinson's disease and began medical treatment. She did well and, so long as she took her medication, had no trouble completing everyday activities—that is, until about six months ago. At that time she began to wake up about two hours earlier than usual because of terrible cramps in her feet. She would try to massage them and sleep again, but usually to no avail. At first the foot cramps woke her up once or twice a week, but then they began to wake her up almost daily. She went to her neurologist, who determined that she was experiencing wearing-off dystonia and prescribed her a longer-acting form of carbidopa/levodopa (levodopa is a medication that is converted to dopamine in the brain) to take at bedtime. Elena found that the new medication relieved the foot cramps, and she was able to sleep through the night once again.*

## Other Symptoms

The nonmotor signs and symptoms of Parkinson's disease are numerous and not as well understood as the motor difficulties. These include cognitive abnormalities, sleep disturbance, urinary incontinence, depression, anxiety, hallucinations, and delusions.

## Cognitive Abnormalities

The issue of whether one's memory and thought process will remain intact is a major concern to men and women with Parkinson's disease as well as to their friends and family. For the most part, people with Parkinson's disease retain their ability to reason, think, and remember events and conversations. Keep in mind that Janet Reno, former Attorney General of the United States, was diagnosed with Parkinson's disease early in her tenure as a member of President Clinton's cabinet. She was able to lead the Justice Department, without difficulty, until the end of his administration.

As the disease itself progresses, people may notice that their thinking, just like their movements, is slower during "off" periods. An off period is when the levels of dopamine in the brain are at a low point in the medication cycle.

Examples of slower thinking include taking longer to respond to someone in a conversation when "off," or having a hard time concentrating on, say, a newspaper article or a book. *Bradyphrenia* is the term used to describe this slow thought process.

It is important to remember that bradyphrenia is distinct from dementia. Bradyphrenia occurs when one is "off." Dementia, by contrast, is the persistent inability to form and retain new memories, retrieve old memories, and perform complex tasks. Dementia is an abnormality in thinking that significantly impairs someone's ability to function on a daily basis. Bradyphrenia, on the other hand, results in slowness in thought or in difficulty finding words without hindering the ability to live or work independently.

## Urinary Incontinence

Urinary incontinence, or the inability to control the flow of urine, is also seen in Parkinson's disease. The severity of urinary dysfunction tends to correlate with the severity of the disease.

Urinary incontinence is not seen early in the course of the disease, and may not be experienced at all by some people with PD. For those who do experience it, however, the most common symptoms of urinary incontinence are increased urinary frequency and increased storage capacity of the bladder because it does not contract to squeeze out the urine as well as it should.

People with Parkinson's disease have a tendency to urinate frequently. This can cause difficulty with sleep. Practical measures to help manage the symptoms include reducing evening fluid intake, emptying the bladder immediately before going to bed, and setting up a bedside commode. Some medications, such as diuretics that are used to control high blood pressure, tend to increase the urge to urinate. In consultation with the prescribing physician, eliminating the use of such medications in the evening may also help. We do not yet understand how Parkinson's disease leads to urinary problems.

## Constipation

Constipation is a frequent complication of Parkinson's disease. Just as the movements of one's limbs slow down, so does the motility of the gastrointestinal tract. With the help of a neurologist, a personalized bowel regimen can be devised to ensure a daily, or every other day, bowel movement. Simple dietary habits, such as drinking six to eight glasses of water daily and eating fruit daily, can help to ensure a regular bowel movement. Medications such as lactulose that are not absorbed by the body and help to retain water in the colon can be prescribed. When water is retained in the colon, the stool that is formed does not get hard and thus is not painful and difficult to excrete. The advantage in establishing a daily regimen to ensure regular bowel movements is that regularity minimizes bloating and discomfort, which can interfere with a person's energy level and overall sense of well-being.

## Sleep Disturbances

Sleep disorders have recently been identified as a common problem in Parkinson's disease. They include trouble falling and staying asleep, vivid dreams, leg or arm cramps, restless legs, and daytime drowsiness. Research on sleep disorders in Parkinson's disease is in its infancy. Below we present a synopsis of the current state of understanding and available treatments for the sleep disorders commonly seen in PD.

In order to understand the sleep abnormalities experienced by people with Parkinson's disease, it is useful to understand what scientific research reveals about a healthy sleep pattern.

To begin, there is no definitive explanation for why we sleep. Although sleep might appear to be a passive state, it is, in fact, a complex, active event involving the brain. Sleep is subdivided into two general states: rapid eye movement (REM) sleep and nonrapid eye movement (NREM) sleep.

REM sleep is the portion of sleep during which there is dreaming and related rapid bursts of eye movement. The function of REM sleep is uncertain, although we know that rats die if they are totally deprived of REM sleep for several weeks. REM sleep is an essential, life-sustaining function.

NREM sleep accounts for about 75 percent of our sleep cycle. It consists of four stages. Stage 1 is the transition from wakefulness to deeper sleep and is the lightest stage of sleep. In young adults, Stage 1 sleep accounts for up to 5 percent of total sleep time. Stage 2 is known as intermediate sleep, and in young adults it accounts for 40 to 50 percent of total sleep time. Stages 3 and 4 sleep are known as deep sleep and typically account for 20 percent of total sleep time in young adults. The function of NREM sleep is also uncertain.

The stages of sleep occur in cycles lasting from 90 to 120 minutes each. Thus, four to five complete cycles occur during a typical night of sleep. During the first half of the night, an individual passes from wakefulness into Stage 1 sleep and then to Stages 2, 3, and 4. Next, Stages 3 and then 2 reappear, after which REM sleep is seen for the first time. During the second half of the night, Stage 2 and REM sleep alternate. (See Figure 6.)

Here is where the problem comes in: In people with sleep disorders, the number of changes from one stage of sleep to another increases and completely disrupts the normal sleep cycle. Adding to that is the aging factor. As we grow older, the amount

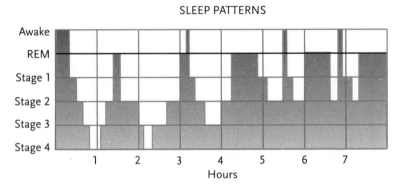

SLEEP PATTERNS

FIGURE 6.    Stages of sleep. A sleeper begins in stage 1, moves through all four stages of sleep, then returns through stages 3 and 2 to a period of REM sleep. For the second half of the night, the sleeper alternates between stage 2 and REM sleep.

Sleep disorders in people with Parkinson's disease are a relatively new area of research. Information regarding the causes and possible treatments of sleep disorders is likely to change markedly in the next few years.

of time that we spend in the deep sleep of Stages 3 and 4 declines while Stage 1 sleep (light sleep) increases.

There is growing evidence that dopamine plays a complex role in the physiology of the sleep-wake cycle. Thus it is not surprising that as control of movement declines in Parkinson's disease, control of sleep declines as well. Studies of people with Parkinson's disease have shown abnormalities in Stages 3 and 4 and in REM sleep.

In normal REM sleep, our muscles are essentially paralyzed. This means that the dreams that occur during REM sleep are not acted out. When an REM disorder exists in Parkinson's disease, however, muscle activity is not inhibited during dreams and excessive motor activity can occur. During truly vivid dreams, the motor activity can be so prominent that a person injures him- or herself or even a bedmate.

A variety of anti-Parkinson drugs can contribute to sleep disruptions. Selegiline (Deprenyl) and amantadine (Symmetrel) are two medications that can increase nighttime wakefulness. Other medications, such as ropinerole (Requip) and pramipexole (Mirapex), have been implicated in excessive daytime sleepiness.

The question of daytime sleepiness in Parkinson's disease is a controversial and complicated one. Some reports have claimed that anti-Parkinson medications are the cause of "sleep attacks" that have resulted in car accidents in otherwise seemingly competent patients. People with Parkinson's disease have many reasons to be sleepy during the day, including disruptions in the normal sleep cycle, as well as depression, which can cause sleepiness in any population.

Some people with Parkinson's disease experience a sleep disorder known as restless legs syndrome. Restless legs syndrome is just what it sounds like—an uncomfortable urge to move one's legs. The urge typically begins or worsens during periods of inactivity and at night. It is relieved by movement. Several studies have attempted to determine whether or not there is an association between restless legs syndrome and Parkinson's disease. Although the methods used in the studies were not optimal, when the data are taken together they suggest that people with Parkinson's disease are more likely to experience restless legs syndrome than the general population. Fortunately, restless legs syndrome can be treated with many of the same medications that are used to treat PD. Thus having both disorders does not mean taking a lot of additional pills.

## Pain and Restlessness

People with Parkinson's disease can experience a variety of sensory symptoms. A sensory symptom is one related to our five senses—touch, sight, hearing, smell, and taste. Pain is an obvious sensory symptom.

At the onset of the disease, when it is mild and only one arm or leg is affected, the first symptom a person with PD experiences is sometimes a persistent, aching pain in that limb. Fortunately, treatment with Parkinson medications typically relieves this pain.

Another sensation may be one of inner restlessness, known as akathisia. This can be a sensation of inner discomfort. It is a generalized feeling of restlessness rather than a pure discomfort in the legs as in restless legs syndrome. Akathisia can be relieved by walking.

## Vision Problems

People with Parkinson's disease may also have problems related to their eyes. One such problem is difficulty reading. Another is dry eye; still another is spasm of the eye lids. Sometimes people literally have to use their fingers to raise their eyelids. Difficulty reading is challenging to evaluate because it can be due to normal aging and the need for eyeglasses, or to the Parkinson's disease, or to both.

The most common problem in people with Parkinson's disease is dry eye and irritation of the surface of the eye caused by the disease-related decrease in the rate of eye blinking. This causes the eyes to become red and irritated and sometimes crusty. Dry eye can be quite uncomfortable, but treatment is relatively easy with artificial tears or a similar medication recommended by an eye doctor.

Spasm of the eyelids, called blepharospasm (*blepharo*, for eyelid; spasm, for uncontrolled muscle contraction) can also be extremely frustrating. Blepharospasm is the uncontrolled contraction of the muscles of the eyelids. It usually begins with excessive blinking and can be triggered by dry eye, bright light, fatigue, or stress. A spasm that becomes so persistent that it interferes with the ability to see can be treated with botulinum toxin injections (commonly known as "Botox"), which weaken the muscles.

An infrequent and usually intermittent problem for some people with Parkinson's disease is double vision, especially at night. Patching one eye can help.

Vision problems in Parkinson's disease should be evaluated and treated by an ophthalmologist. An eye doctor should be included as a member of the treatment team.

### Depression

Depression is so common in Parkinson's disease that we have devoted a long section to it later in the book. The National Parkinson's Foundation reports that about 40 percent of people with Parkinson's disease experience depression. This might seem obvious; after all, it only makes sense that someone with any chronic, debilitating disease would become depressed. But the truth is that depression is more common in Parkinson's disease than in other chronic illnesses. Interestingly, there is even evidence that depression can precede the onset of symptoms of Parkinson's disease. A detailed discussion of depression and other psychological aspects of Parkinson's disease is presented in Chapter 8.

## Making the Diagnosis

When a doctor sees a patient for the first time, it can be difficult to be certain that the proper diagnosis is Parkinson's disease and that the patient does not have one of several other neurodegenerative disorders.

The array of similar-looking disorders are known collectively as the Parkinson's Plus Syndromes and include multiple system atrophy (MSA) and progressive supranuclear palsy (PSP). MSA is distinguished by the presence of symptoms that include urinary incontinence, reduced sweating, and a significant drop in blood pressure when a person stands up. A characteristic of PSP is the inability to exercise voluntarily movement of the eyes. Another feature of PSP is a marked change in personality; family members are quick to note apathy or inappropriate laughter. Despite these guiding principles, they still turn out to be crude criteria for making a diagnosis within a group of poorly understood diseases.

Adding to the difficulty is a form of dementia that has some of the motor features of Parkinson's disease. This condition is known as Diffuse Lewy Body Disease (DLBD) and consists of a marked decline in intellectual function, visual hallucinations, and signs of bradykinesia, rigidity, and possibly rest tremor. DLBD is a disease that has been differentiated from other forms of dementia and formally studied only recently. As a result, information regarding the prevalence of DLBD is limited at this time.

Conventional laboratory investigations typically do not contribute to the diagnosis or management of Parkinson's disease. Computed tomography (CT) and magnetic resonance imaging (MRI) scans of the brain, which provide detailed anatomic information about the brain, do not reveal any consistent abnormalities in people with Parkinson's disease. An experimental imaging technique called positron emission tomography (PET) may be more helpful. PET examines blood flow and metabolism in the brain. Another experimental imaging technique is single photon emission computed tomography (SPECT). SPECT is used to examine blood flow in the brain and the activity of various receptors in the brain. At this time, both PET and SPECT are only performed as part of a research study and are not standard clinical tools.

## Questions the Doctor Might Ask

Making a diagnosis of Parkinson's disease can be difficult, even for an experienced physician. Thus any symptoms that the patient and family members or friends describe for the doctor can be especially helpful. Patients are sometimes unaware of signs—such as stooped posture, slow movement, or changes in facial expression—that other people notice. On a visit to the doctor, it is very important to have a thoughtful and observant companion accompany the patient.

The following are some questions that a doctor typically asks a patient when considering the diagnosis of Parkinson's disease. We list the questions here to give the person who is about to visit the doctor a chance to think about the answers. It is often helpful to mull over answers in advance, and to have family members report what they have noticed:

- Are you walking more slowly?
- Do you take longer to get ready in the morning?
- Do you have trouble turning in bed?
- Do you cough or choke while eating or drinking?
- Do you take longer to handle utensils and eat a meal?
- Do you have a tendency to lean or fall backward?
- Do friends and family complain that you are more difficult to understand on the telephone?
- Do coworkers, friends, or family members complain that your handwriting has become more difficult to interpret?
- Are you having daily, or every other day, bowel movements, or are you having trouble with constipation?
- Have you noticed a tendency to drool?

A yes or no answer does not necessarily indicate Parkinson's disease or one of the Parkinson's Plus Syndromes.

## What Does a Diagnosis of PD Mean?

So you or someone important in your life has been diagnosed with Parkinson's disease. As you gather information, you will undoubtedly have many questions. We hope that the questions and answers below will provide some important information to help you begin dealing with the presence of Parkinson's disease in your life.

### WILL HAVING PARKINSON'S DISEASE SHORTEN MY LIFE?

Because of the rapid pace of research into treatment for Parkinson's disease, there is currently no clear answer to this question. Keep in mind that each case of Parkinson's disease is different. For people whose symptoms do not progress rapidly, who begin to experience symptoms at an older age, and who remain in one of the first three stages of the disease for many years, Parkinson's disease is not likely to shorten the lifespan.

### IS IT OKAY TO DRIVE?

A diagnosis of Parkinson's disease does not, in and of itself, mean that a person must give up the car keys and never be alone again. Keep in mind that the symptoms and severity of Parkinson's disease vary tremendously from person to person, so it is important to talk to your doctor and develop a treatment and lifestyle plan that is tailored to your personal needs and circumstances.

The biggest concern surrounding driving is whether the reaction time of a person with Parkinson's disease is quick enough. Because one of the primary symptoms of Parkinson's disease is slowness of movement, the question arises about the driver's ability to hit the brakes or steer quickly in an emergency. Although no one likes the idea of giving up their independence, it is important to remember that safety—yours and that of others on the road—must be your first concern.

Laws about who may drive vary from state to state. Most states have programs for evaluating drivers to determine who can drive safely. If you have any doubts, contact your local department of motor vehicles. Ask about the rules and whether programs exist for evaluating driving skills. Some rehabilitation hospitals and clinics offer programs to evaluate the ability to drive. These programs typically charge a fee not covered by insurance.

### WHAT ABOUT WORK?

Work should be continued whenever possible. Because the symptoms of Parkinson's disease vary so much from one person to another, it is impossible to predict how long a specific person can continue to work. Keep in mind that many people are able to retire at the age they had originally planned before being diagnosed with Parkinson's disease. Getting a diagnosis of PD does not automatically mean early retirement.

Continuing to work will not make the course of the disease any worse. If an individual with Parkinson's disease travels frequently for work, there is no reason to cut back on that activity, either. If you are a spouse or partner who travels frequently for business, you should not feel compelled to stay at home. The important thing to remember is that with the range of treatments available today, the person with Parkinson's disease can continue to lead a full and active life.

*Tara works as a manager in research and development at a chemical company. Three years ago, at the age of fifty-eight, she was diagnosed with Parkinson's disease. Her primary symptoms were a stiffness in the right arm and worsening handwriting. Her secretary had begun to complain that her handwriting was difficult to read, at which point Tara realized she needed to see her doctor. Once she began medical treatment, the stiffness greatly improved. Although her handwriting was still difficult to read, she began using the computer more and e-mailed her secretary, rather than giving her handwritten notes.*

*Philip is fifty-one and drives an armored truck. He was diagnosed with Parkinson's disease six months ago, when his internist noted that he had a resting tremor in his left hand. Philip saw a neurologist, who confirmed the diagnosis. Because the tremor completely disappears when he moves his arm for a specific purpose, such as turning on the high beams in his truck, and because Philip himself does not think the tremor is affecting him, he is not taking any Parkinson medications. His wife, however, is worried about his safety at work. Philip did not want to tell his employers about the diagnosis for fear that he would lose his job. His wife, however, convinced him to call the Department of Motor Vehicles and arrange for a road test. Philip paid for the test himself, and was relieved to find that he was driving well enough to pass. Equipped with this information, both he and his wife feel much better about his continuing in his current job.*

### DOES STRESS OR EXCITEMENT INTENSIFY SYMPTOMS?

Yes. Any type of stress or excitement can intensify tremor and the other symptoms of Parkinson's disease. People often think of stress as something that affects them emotionally. Physical stress, like a cold or the flu, can have the same effect as emotional stress. *Stress does not, however, make the course of the disease any worse.* There is no way to determine what the course of Parkinson's disease will be in a particular individual.

It is especially important for family members to keep in mind these facts about stress and excitement. There is no reason to keep bad news from a family member who has Parkinson's disease, because any effect the stress might have on symptoms will be temporary. If anything, family relationships may become strained if information or news that was routinely shared before the diagnosis is suddenly withheld.

### IS IT OKAY FOR A PERSON WITH PARKINSON'S DISEASE TO DRINK ALCOHOLIC BEVERAGES?

An occasional cocktail or glass of wine or beer with a meal is usually fine, depending on the specific medications being taken.

The best thing to do is discuss the issue with the physician or physicians who prescribe the medications.

### CAN WE STILL TRAVEL?

Yes. People with Parkinson's disease can and should continue to live a full life. If you enjoy traveling, then by all means do so. A good source of information regarding services and accessibility for those with diminished mobility is the Internet site www.access-able.com. This website contains accounts of actual travel experiences to different cities, all over the world, as well as a list of travel agents who specialize in travel for those with special needs.

Be sure to leave town with more than enough medication so that there is no chance you can run out. Your physician and pharmacist should work with you to ensure that the medication is adequate for a comfortable trip. If medications should run out, rest assured that drugs for Parkinson's disease are available in hospitals and pharmacies throughout the world. It is a good idea to write down the names (generic names and brand names) and doses of all medications and store them in a secure place in case you need to purchase more while you are away.

### WHAT ABOUT BEING ALONE AT HOME, OR ANYWHERE ELSE?

There is no reason to change your habits. This applies to the person with Parkinson's disease as well as to family members. Continue to work, exercise, and pursue hobbies just like before. Family members should understand that being overprotective often leads to resentment and tension in the relationship. Leaving a loved one home alone will not adversely affect the disease. It is important for everyone to maintain independence.

*Jim is seventy years old and was just diagnosed with Parkinson's disease. His wife, Maria, had noticed that he was slower in walking and getting dressed and urged him to go to the doctor. Once they were given the diagnosis, Jim began medication and felt that he was fine. Maria, however, became scared to leave him alone.*

*Since his retirement at the age of sixty-two, Jim had been in the daily habit of taking an early morning walk by himself. He enjoyed walking through his neighborhood at 6:00 A.M., before the daily rush of his neighbors heading off to school and work. Maria, however, was not a morning person and typically did not get up and out of the house until 10:00 or 11:00 A.M. Maria first tried to get up early to accompany Jim on his walks, but she did not like exercising in the morning and Jim found that her presence and persistent conversation made the walks less enjoyable. After a week of joint walks, Maria realized that Jim was perfectly steady and safe by himself. She also loathed getting up at such an early hour. Maria reverted to her usual schedule, and Jim was relieved to be able to enjoy his morning walks on his own.*

### WHAT HAPPENS WITH BLADDER AND BOWEL CONTROL?

Many people with Parkinson's disease experience constipation. This is because the motility of the intestines decreases. There are many ways to ensure a bowel movement daily or every other day. These methods, which are referred to as bowel regimens, typically include one or more of the following: exercise, dietary changes, adequate intake of fluids, and oral or rectal medication, if necessary. Each bowel regimen is unique, but it is important to know that regular bowel movements can be maintained in people who have Parkinson's disease.

*Jill was diagnosed with Parkinson's disease two years ago. Her main symptom was a rest tremor in the left arm that made her arm feel sore by the end of the day. The tremor was fairly well controlled with medication, and so the ache in her arm was minimal. But Jill was experiencing more and more difficulty with constipation. At first, she found that she could maintain a daily bowel movement by drinking two full glasses of water between every meal and eating fruit with breakfast and lunch. Recently, however, she has been moving her bowels only every second or third day, and she feels bloated and un-comfortable on the other days. When she saw her neurologist, they discussed this problem and she began taking lactulose twice a day. The combination of prescription medication, fruit, and water did the trick, and Jill resumed her schedule of daily bowel movements.*

Some people with Parkinson's disease do suffer from abnormalities in bladder function. For example, they may have difficulty starting or stopping urination. Urinary problems can be due to the Parkinson's disease itself, the medications taken to treat Parkinson's disease, or a combination of both. Patients experiencing urinary difficulties should discuss the problem with their neurologist, who may suggest they be evaluated by a urologist as well.

## Standards for Staging Parkinson's Disease

Patients and their family members often ask about the stages of Parkinson's disease. They want to know how far along they or their loved ones are in the course of the disease. Parkinson's disease is progressive, meaning that symptoms worsen over time, but it progresses at a different rate in every patient. PD produces a variable constellation of signs and symptoms in any given stage. The length of time that one person may spend in a particular stage is difficult, if not impossible, to predict.

Parkinson's disease can be staged, thanks to Drs. Margaret Hoehn and Melvin Yahr, who in 1967 introduced a 6-point rating scale that has been widely adopted. The scale ranks symptoms on a magnitude of 0–5, with 0 indicating no visible symptoms of disease and 5 indicating the most troubling symptoms. Doctors stage an individual patient's disease in order to have an objective measure of how that person fares from year to year. The scale also allows comparison of a patient's response to medication. Keep in mind that this staging system was developed at a time when medications were not available for the symptomatic treatment of Parkinson's disease. Today, thanks to the numerous medical and surgical treatments available, many patients with Parkinson's disease never reach stage 5.

The Hoehn and Yahr Scale rates mobility. Other scales measure additional conditions that many people with Parkinson's disease share. One such scale is the Unified Parkinson's Disease Rating Scale (UPDRS). It rates four areas: mentation (mental activity), behavior, and mood; activities of daily living; motor skills (mobility); and complications of therapy. The doctor or an assistant administers a questionnaire that covers topics ranging from dressing and hygiene to symptoms of anxiety. The total UPDRS score is a sum of the score on each of the four sections. The score can range from 0, meaning no disability, to a maximum of 199, representing total disability.

Clinicians around the world use the UPDRS as a means of monitoring the course of Parkinson's disease and the response to medications. Keep in mind that these scales are not perfect measures of disease; nor does the number generated by the scales take the place of the details of symptoms experienced by an individual with Parkinson's disease. One person may feel better after beginning treatment with a particular medication, but his or her score on the UPDRS may not improve. The primary purpose of these scales is to facilitate clinical research.

The Hoehn and Yahr and UPDRS scales were developed and are used specifically for those with Parkinson's disease. In contrast, the Schwab and England Activities of Daily Living Scale was developed to examine a person's ability to live independently regardless of the underlying disease. It is scored in 10 percent increments, from 100 percent, indicating that a person is independent and able to do all chores without slowness, difficulty, or impairment, to 0 percent, representing the most difficult circumstances. The Hoehn and Yahr Scale, portions of each section of the UPDRS, and the Schwab and England Activities of Daily Living Scale are shown below.

*Tip:* Use these scales to become acquainted with Parkinson's disease. Use them as a reminder to learn as much as possible about the disorder and about the abundant resources that are available for coping.

### HOEHN AND YAHR STAGING OF PARKINSON'S DISEASE

0. Stage Zero, no visible symptoms of Parkinson's disease
1. Stage One
   1. Signs and symptoms on one side only
   2. Symptoms mild
   3. Symptoms inconvenient but not disabling
   4. Usually presents with tremor of one limb
   5. Friends have noticed changes in posture, locomotion, and facial expression
2. Stage Two
   1. Symptoms are bilateral (on both sides of the body)
   2. Minimal disability
   3. Posture and gait affected
3. Stage Three
   1. Significant slowing of body movements
   2. Early impairment of equilibrium on walking or standing
   3. Generalized dysfunction that is moderately severe
4. Stage Four
   1. Severe symptoms
   2. Can still walk to a limited extent
   3. Rigidity and bradykinesia
   4. No longer able to live alone

5. Tremor may be less than earlier stages

5. Stage Five

   1. Cachectic stage (cachexia is a state of malnutrition and wasting. It may occur in many chronic diseases)

   2. Invalidism complete

   3. Cannot stand or walk

   4. Requires constant nursing care

## UNIFIED PARKINSON DISEASE RATING SCALE (UPDRS)

  I. Mentation, Behavior, Mood

   *Intellectual Impairment*

    0. None

    1. Mild (consistent forgetfulness with partial recollection of events with no other difficulties)

    2. Moderate memory loss with disorientation and moderate difficulty handling complex problems

    3. Severe memory loss with disorientation to time and often place, severe impairment in handling problems

    4. Severe memory loss, orientation only to person, unable to make judgments or solve problems, can't be left alone at all

   *Thought Disorder*

    0. None

    1. Vivid dreaming

    2. "Benign" hallucinations with insight retained

    3. Occasional to frequent hallucinations or delusions without insight; could interfere with daily activities

    4. Persistent hallucinations, delusions or florid psychosis; not able to care for self

   *Motivation/Initiative*

    0. Normal

    1. Less assertive than usual, more passive

    2. Loss of initiative or disinterest in elective activities

    3. Loss of initiative or disinterest in day-to-day (routine) activities

    4. Withdrawn, complete loss of motivation

*Depression*

    0. Not present

    1. Periods of sadness or guilt greater than normal, never sustained for days or weeks

    2. Sustained depression for $>/=$ 1 week

    3. Sustained depression with vegetative symptoms (insomnia, anorexia, weight loss)

    4. Sustained depression with vegetative symptoms and suicidal thoughts or intent

II. Activities of Daily Living

*Speech*

    0. Normal

    1. Mildly affected; no difficulty being understood

    2. Moderately affected; sometimes asked to repeat statements

    3. Severely affected; frequently asked to repeat statements

    4. Unintelligible most of the time

*Swallowing*

    0. Normal

    1. Rare choking

    2. Occasional choking

    3. Requires soft food

    4. Requires nasogastric tube or gastrostomy feeding

*Handwriting*

    0. Normal

    1. Slightly small or slow

    2. Moderately slow or small; all words small but legible

    3. Severely affected, not all words legible

    4. Majority of words illegible

*Cutting Food and Handling Utensils*
- 0. Normal
- 1. Somewhat slow and clumsy but no help needed
- 2. Can cut most foods, although clumsy and slow; some help needed
- 3. Food must be cut by someone, but can still feed self slowly
- 4. Needs to be fed

*Dressing*
- 0. Normal
- 1. Somewhat slow, but no help needed
- 2. Occasional help with buttons or arms in sleeves
- 3. Considerable help required, but can do some things alone
- 4. Helpless

*Turning in Bed and Adjusting Bedclothes*
- 0. Normal
- 1. Somewhat slow and clumsy, but no help needed
- 2. Can turn alone or adjust sheets, but with great difficulty
- 3. Can initiate attempt, but cannot turn or adjust sheets alone
- 4. Helpless

*Falling (Unrelated to Freezing)*
- 0. None
- 1. Rare falling
- 2. Occasionally falls; less than once daily
- 3. Falls an average of once daily
- 4. Falls more than once daily

*Freezing when Walking*
- 0. None
- 1. Rare freezing when walking; may have start hesitation
- 2. Occasional freezing when walking

3. Frequent freezing, occasionally falls because of freezing
4. Frequently falls because of freezing

*Walking*

0. Normal
1. Mild difficulty; may not swing arms or may tend to drag leg
2. Moderate difficulty, but requires little or no assistance
3. Severe disturbance of walking; requires assistance
4. Cannot walk at all, even with assistance

*Tremor*

Examined in both the right arm and the left arm; each arm is given a score according to the following scale

0. Absent
1. Slight and infrequently present; not bothersome to the patient
2. Moderate; bothersome to patient
3. Severe; interferes with many activities
4. Marked; interferes with most activities

III. Motor Exam

*Speech*

0. Normal
1. Slight loss of expression, diction, volume
2. Monotone, slurred but understandable
3. Marked impairment, difficult to understand
4. Unintelligible

*Facial Expression*

0. Normal
1. Slight hypomimia, could be "poker face" in someone without PD
2. Slight but definite abnormal diminution in expression
3. Masked or fixed face with complete loss of expression

*Tremor at Rest*

Rated in the face and each limb (right arm, left arm, right leg, and left leg)

0. Absent
1. Slight and infrequent
2. Mild and present most of time
3. Moderate and present most of time
4. Marked and present most of time

*Rigidity*

Tested in the neck and each limb (right arm, left arm, right leg, and left leg)

0. Absent
1. Slight or only with activation
2. Mild/moderate
3. Marked, full range of motion
4. Severe

*Gait*

0. Normal
1. Walks slowly, may shuffle with short steps, no gait acceleration or propulsion
2. Walks with difficulty, little or no assistance, some gait acceleration, short steps or propulsion
3. Severe disturbance, needs frequent assistance
4. Cannot walk

*Body Bradykinesia/Hypokinesia*

0. None
1. Minimal slowness, could be normal, deliberate character
2. Mild slowness and poverty of movement, definitely abnormal, or decreased amplitude of movement
3. Moderate slowness, poverty, or small amplitude
4. Marked slowness, poverty, or amplitude

*Complications of Therapy (in Week prior to Visit)*

Dyskinesias

What proportion of the waking day are dyskinesias present?

0. None
1. 1–25 percent of the day
2. 26–50 percent of the day
3. 51–75 percent of the day
4. 76–100 percent of the day

### SCHWAB AND ENGLAND ACTIVITIES OF DAILY LIVING SCALE

*100 percent:* Completely independent and essentially normal. The individual is able to do all chores without impairment and is unaware of any difficulty.

*90 percent:* Completely independent. The individual is able to do all chores with some degree of difficulty and may take twice as long. The individual is beginning to be aware of difficulty.

*80 percent:* Completely independent in most chores but does take twice as long to complete them. The individual is conscious of difficulty and slowness.

*70 percent:* Not completely independent. The individual has more difficulty with chores and may take three to four times longer to complete some of them. Must spend a large part of the day on chores.

*60 percent:* There is some dependency. The individual can do most chores, but exceedingly slowly and with much effort. Some chores are impossible to complete without help.

*50 percent:* More dependent. The individual has difficulty with everything.

*40 percent:* Very dependent. The individual can assist with all chores, but can complete few alone.

*30 percent:* The individual can, with effort, do a few chores alone or begin them alone. Much help is needed.

*20 percent:* The individual is unable to complete any chore alone. Can be a slight help with some chores. Severe invalid.

*10 percent:* Totally dependent, helpless. Complete invalid.

*0 percent:* Vegetative functions such as swallowing, bladder and bowel functions are not functioning. Bedridden.

Although being rated according to these scales may seem tedious and time-consuming, the tests are valuable and do not take long to complete. The UPDRS, in particular, has been a great aid to researchers who are testing new drugs for treating the symptoms of Parkinson's disease.

# 3

## Risk Factors

You may be wondering what put your relative or friend at risk for Parkinson's disease. Why Jack or Maria or Jennifer or Manuel? Why not Roberto or Dave or Cheryl?

People sometimes ask about risk because they want to understand their role in causing Parkinson's disease or their ability to prevent it from happening to other family members.

First, no one causes another person to come down with Parkinson's disease. Second, PD so rarely affects more than one person in a family that it is pointless to worry that it may occur in multiple family members.

That having been said, the question of risk factors for Parkinson's disease is still a good one, and researchers are looking for answers. A risk factor is defined as something that may increase someone's chance of developing a disease. For example, cigarette smoking is a risk factor for cardiac disease.

Scientists have been trying for years to identify behaviors, toxins, genetics, or any other risk factors for Parkinson's disease. A few possible risk factors have emerged:

- genetics
- environmental agents
- age

Studies looking at the distribution and causes of Parkinson's disease indicate that a combination of genetic and environmental factors could play a role in the development of the disease. Age is considered a risk factor because the vast majority of people who develop Parkinson's disease are well past middle age; the average age of onset is sixty.

## Genetics

Genetics is the study of heredity and how it varies from person to person. A gene is a specific portion of DNA, on a specific chromosome, that contains the instructions for the production of a specific protein.

Proteins are made up of individual units, known as amino acids. The DNA of each gene is similar to a cooking recipe; it instructs the cell as to which amino acids should be put together, and in what order, to produce a specific protein. Each human inherits a pair of genes for every protein produced in his or her body, with one gene coming from each parent. These genes become activated, in different cells and at different times during development, and direct the cell to produce a particular protein.

In the vast majority of cases, a specific protein produced in one person is the same as that protein produced in another person. This is because the protein is vital for our bodies to function properly. In some instances, however, one or both of the genes that are inherited contain a mutation. A mutation refers to a change in a specific gene, resulting in a difference in the protein it produces. Sometimes these mutations result in a protein that no longer functions. In other instances, a mutation results in a protein that functions in an abnormal way.

Mutations in several different genes have been identified in some families with Parkinson's disease. Each family, as discussed in detail below, has a mutation in a single gene that results in the production of an abnormal protein. To date, mutations in one of three different genes have been identified.

*What about My Children?*

There is no reason to worry that because you have been diagnosed with Parkinson's disease your children are at risk. In a
handful of families, researchers have identified genes that cause
PD. In these families, some children and not others develop the
disease. In the vast majority of cases, however, Parkinson's disease develops in an individual with no clear inheritance pattern.
If you're worried about inheritance, discuss your concerns with
your doctor and perhaps a genetic counselor. Genetic counsel-
ors are health care professionals with specialized graduate degrees and experience in the areas of medical genetics and counseling. They work as part of a health care team and provide
information and support to families who have members with
genetic disorders, as well as to families who may be at risk for
a variety of inherited conditions.

## Families with Gene-Related Parkinson's Disease

In very few families around the world, an unusual number of
members have Parkinson's disease, and it is obvious that the disease has been passed down from one generation to the next. The
affected family members, researchers have discovered, share a
mutation in a particular gene. This mutation causes an error in
the production of a certain protein that influences the brain.

Researchers have identified a number of different gene mutations for Parkinson's disease. The first was found in several generations of an Italian family, referred to by scientists and physicians as the Contursi kindred. The family originated in the town
of Contursi, in the Salerno province of Italy. Sixty family members, over five generations, are known to have had Parkinson's
disease.

The cause of Parkinson's disease in the Contursi family turns

> ## What Did I Do to Get Parkinson's Disease?
>
> The symptoms of Parkinson's disease are the result of the loss of brain cells that produce a chemical called dopamine. The critical event, the one that causes the dopamine-producing brain cells to die, is not known. Despite extensive research, no lifestyle factors have been identified that increase a person's risk of getting Parkinson's disease. So there is nothing that an individual should or should not do to decrease the risk of Parkinson's disease. It is important to remember that you did nothing to get PD.

out to be a mutation in the gene that produces a protein called alpha-synuclein. The gene mutation causes one change in the protein's amino acid composition. Scientists do not know how this production of a mutated alpha-synuclein protein causes Parkinson's disease. This particular genetic defect is extremely rare and has only been found in a few families.

A different problem involving the alpha-synuclein protein has been identified in another large family in which several members have been diagnosed with early-onset Parkinson's disease (symptoms begin before the age of forty). Neurologists at the Mayo Clinic in Minnesota first evaluated members of this family in 1920 and have continued to study healthy and affected descendants for more than eighty years. In 2004, with the introduction of highly sophisticated techniques for identifying genes and genetic abnormalities, scientists at the National Institutes of Health discovered the probable genetic cause—affected family members carry four copies of the normal gene for alpha-synuclein instead of the normal two copies. It appears that in this family, having an excess of the normal alpha-synuclein protein results in Parkinson's disease.

Early-onset Parkinson's disease has also been linked to the

mutation of a second protein, called parkin. In a survey of seventy-three families with early-onset Parkinson's disease, more than half produced an abnormal parkin protein. As with alpha-synuclein, the function of the normal parkin protein is not well understood, and we don't know why production of an abnormal parkin protein results in Parkinson's disease.

A mutation in a third protein, called by the nearly unpronounceable name of ubiquitin carboxy-terminal hydrolase L1 (UCH-L1), has been identified in a German family in which multiple members have Parkinson's disease. An interesting finding in this family tells us a lot about risk factors and how they can be influenced by other events. It turns out that only some of the family members who have the mutation in UCH-L1 have Parkinson's disease. Others are disease-free, revealing that having the mutation does not guarantee that the disease will develop. Other factors obviously come into play. UCH-L1 is involved in the processing and breakdown of proteins within brain cells. A defect in UCH-L1 may lead to an accumulation of proteins within the cells that may cause their death. The exact mechanism by which a mutation in UCH-L1 results in PD is uncertain.

## Environment

Research has suggested that substances in our environment might increase the risk of Parkinson's disease. For the first indication that this might be the case, we can look back to 1817, when James Parkinson wrote the first unequivocal description of Parkinson's disease. Some researchers believe that the date of the report is evidence of an environmental cause for PD: the case was reported during the Industrial Revolution, a time when huge amounts of pollutants were being released into the air through the burning of coal.

Industrial byproducts that have been implicated as possible contributors to Parkinson's disease include copper, lead, manganese, mercury, and zinc. We say "implicated" because a causal relationship between a specific metal and the incidence of Parkinson's disease has been studied infrequently and only in small populations, which makes it difficult to argue for a definite cause-and-effect relationship.

One unfortunate event does, though, demonstrate that "Parkinson-like" symptoms can be attributed to external circumstances. The event occurred in 1982 in the Bay Area of California and involved heroin users who had injected themselves with a synthetic narcotic. The drug turned out to contain a powerful and damaging chemical referred to as MPTP. The compound killed nerve cells in the same part of the brain that is affected in people with Parkinson's disease and caused sudden, severe, and permanent symptoms that looked like Parkinson's disease.

Other environmental risk factors that have been implicated in the development of Parkinson's disease are pesticides (substances for destroying or controlling animal pests or plants) and herbicides (substances specifically meant to kill unwanted plant growth). Several studies have associated pesticide and herbicide use with an increased risk of Parkinson's disease. However, the relationship between exposure to these chemicals and the development of PD is poorly understood. Specifically, studies of the effects of pesticides and herbicides involve the short-term exposure of rodents to relatively high levels of the chemical in question. It is difficult to then translate the results of this work to real-world exposure.

The relationship between environmental exposure and Parkinson's disease is extremely complicated, and research based on experience with MPTP and herbicides and pesticides shows just how difficult it can be to interpret findings. For example, researchers have focused on the effect of herbicides and pesticides that have a chemical structure similar to that of MPTP. One example is an herbicide called paraquat. Adult mice that were exposed to paraquat as newborns had decreased brain dopamine levels. The mice did not, however, display signs of Parkinson's disease, and, since most newborn babies are protected from exposure to herbicides and pesticides, it is not clear what this finding in mice means in terms of the development of Parkinson's disease in adult humans. To date, no herbicide or pesticide has been identified as clearly causing Parkinson's disease. Hence, there is no evidence to suggest that the use of herbicides on your lawn or garden, provided that you follow the precautions recommended by the manufacturer to minimize exposure, increases the risk of developing Parkinson's disease.

## Age

The most definitive risk factor for Parkinson's disease is aging. Studies show that the prevalence of Parkinson's disease increases up to the ninth decade (ages eighty to eighty-nine) of life. Reliable information regarding the prevalence of Parkinson's disease beyond the ninth decade is not available. This relationship between PD and old age correlates with normal changes in brain chemistry related to growing older. The number of cell receptors for dopamine, the neurotransmitter that is present in insufficient quantities in the brains of people with Parkinson's disease, decreases as we age. This has been shown using a sophisticated medical imaging technique called PET (positron emission tomography). PET allows researchers to see the brain as it responds to various stimuli.

## Reducing Risk

Now that we have discussed risk factors for Parkinson's disease, what about factors that may *reduce* the risk of developing Parkin-

*Is There Anything I Should Not Do?*

No. It is important to remember that there are no lifestyle factors that play a role in the development or course of Parkinson's disease. There is no reason to feel guilty about previous actions, and there is no reason to stop doing the things you enjoy.

son's disease? In a strange twist, research suggests that cigarette smoking and coffee consumption may be two such factors.

Several large studies have identified caffeine consumption and smoking as possible factors that protect against Parkinson's disease. In one study of nearly 14,000 residents of a retirement community in southern California, Parkinson's disease was found to be significantly less common among coffee drinkers and smokers than among those who didn't smoke or drink caffeine.[1] Again, we do not know why. The findings have been supported in studies of rodents: caffeine was found to have a beneficial effect on dopamine signaling in the brain; nicotine, the addictive component of cigarettes, also appeared to promote the effects of dopamine in the brain. This news is not meant as encouragement to smoke cigarettes or increase coffee consumption. There is no evidence to support the notion that someone diagnosed with Parkinson's disease would benefit from cigarette smoking, but there is ample evidence that smoking increases the risk of lung cancer, heart disease, and other medical conditions. Other lifestyle factors, such as level of exercise, diet, and weight, have not been shown to affect a person's risk of developing Parkinson's disease.

# 4

## Treatment

Until the introduction of levodopa in the 1960s, there was no effective treatment for Parkinson's disease.[1] Today, getting good treatment should not be too challenging. In addition to medications, there are many support organizations designed to help people cope with the disease. Such groups are staffed by compassionate and knowledgeable individuals prepared to help patients and families. The Internet is a good resource for finding support organizations, as is your local library. Health care providers who treat Parkinson's disease should also know where patients and families can get information, if not right there in the doctor's office.

If you live in a city or large town, you may have many choices of caregivers, making it difficult to select from what could be dozens or even hundreds of professionals. Take Baltimore, Maryland, as an example. The city's telephone directory lists nearly three hundred physical therapists or physical therapy practices. (Physical therapy, or PT, is one of the treatments recommended for people with Parkinson's disease.) How do you find out which practices focus on patients with neurodegenerative disorders, and which would suit you best? Searching for the care that's right for you takes patience and research. Begin by discussing with your friend or family member who has Parkinson's disease just how involved he or she would like you to be in treatment decisions and activities. Some patients and families thrive on managing the disease together. Others find that it leads to too much togetherness and tension, which can create frustration and even hostility. Be patient; it may take a little time to arrive at the right level of involvement, and that level may fluctuate from time to time.

## The First Step

The first step after diagnosis, typically, is to find a neurologist. A neurologist is a medical doctor specially trained to care for patients who have a disease of the nervous system (the brain, spinal cord, and nerves that supply muscles and other structures of the body). Some neurologists even have additional training in the area of movement disorders. Some go even further and focus mainly on Parkinson's disease. Many large medical institutions house a center that specializes exclusively in movement disorders or Parkinson's disease.

Your family physician will probably give you a list of neurologists from which to choose. Take steps to ensure that the prospective neurologist is right for you. Ask, for example, in what field the doctor is board certified. Board certification indicates that the physician has passed a comprehensive exam given by other doctors in his or her specialty. Check with the neurologist's office staff to ensure that they can process claims from your health insurance company. Choose a doctor whose age and sex suits you. In addition to your personal physician, members of Parkinson's disease support groups can be a good source of references.

Now that you or someone you love has been diagnosed, what kinds of treatment are available and recommended for patients with Parkinson's disease? Current treatment for Parkinson's disease falls into five major categories:

- physical therapy
- occupational therapy

*Is Exercise OK?*

Absolutely! Exercise is good for overall health and for maintaining flexibility, strength, balance, endurance, and mobility. Exercise does not worsen Parkinson's disease.

Before beginning an exercise program, consult your doctor to make sure there are no exercises you should avoid for any health reason. Then, consult a physical therapist to establish an exercise regimen that is healthy and appropriate for you. Begin any exercise routine slowly. Build up as your strength improves.

Keep in mind that a healthy exercise program does not require expensive equipment or membership at an exclusive gym. A comprehensive exercise routine can be followed using simple equipment or no equipment at all. For example, stretching calf muscles by pushing against a wall is a great way to promote flexibility of the legs. Standing with one's back to the wall and slowly bending at the knees helps strengthen the muscles of the buttocks and thighs without the risk of a fall. Holding onto the kitchen counter while standing on one leg is a simple method of improving balance, and taking a daily walk or riding a stationary bike is a great way to build endurance.

- speech therapy
- medical treatment
- surgical treatment

Physical and occupational therapies focus on mobility, the use of adaptive equipment, and safety in the home, workplace, and community. These therapies are designed to improve a person's motor function as well as muscle strength and tone, and help maintain an adequate range of motion in the joints. (See Figure 7.) Physical, occupational, and speech therapies work best when

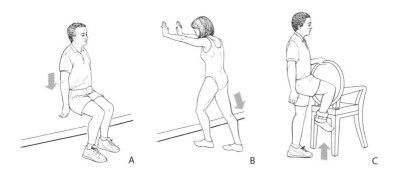

FIGURE 7.    Simple stretching and strengthening exercises. 7A.) Modified squats: Stand with your back against the wall and look straight
ahead. Keep your feet shoulder-width apart and 18 to 24 inches in
front of your torso. Slowly bend at the knees until you are in a "sitting" position. 7B.) Runner's stretch: Lean against the wall, keeping
your arms at shoulder height, and stretch each calf in turn.
7C.) Quadriceps strengthening: At the kitchen counter or dining
room table, stand with a chair in front of you. Hold on to the edge of
the tabletop and the top of the chair and look straight ahead, to maintain balance. Bend and lift first one knee then the other. After working
on this for several weeks, you may add a small (1 to 3 lb.) ankle
weight, if your physical therapist and physicians approve the use of
weights.


drug regimens are effective. Thus, it is helpful to schedule therapy sessions for one to two hours after the last dose of medication, when drug levels are at their peak in the brain.

   In addition to gaining physically from the various therapies, a
person who is involved in treatment gains a measure of control
over the symptoms of the disease and satisfaction in being able
to manage some of its aspects. As you will read later in this
book, people with Parkinson's disease often experience psychological symptoms, which are generally easier to manage if the
patient is leading an active and involved life. Even though Parkinson's disease causes most patients to become increasingly

slow in their movements and muted in their speech, these therapies will help individuals maximize their abilities.

All five major categories of treatment are described in detail in
this chapter.

## Physical Therapy

As we discussed in earlier chapters, Parkinson's disease is progressive, meaning that symptoms continue to worsen over time.
Because physical therapy improves motor skills, people with
Parkinson's disease can benefit from physical therapy throughout the course of their illness.

Physical therapists are licensed health care professionals who
teach a variety of strategies for coping with impairments or
disabilities. These strategies help people move more easily,
minimize disability, and retain independence. Parkinson's disease centers usually employ physical therapists who specialize in treating Parkinson's patients. The advantage of working
with these specialists is that they know Parkinson's disease and
how the symptoms are affected by medication and other treatments.

Ideally, physical therapy should include sessions in which the
therapist works with the patient in his or her home and community. Particular emphasis should be placed on easing access and
mobility in the bathroom and kitchen in order to avoid the risk
of injury. Around the neighborhood, emphasis should be on
safety at street crossings (including negotiating curbs) and on
getting in and out of cars and buses. When getting out of a vehi-
cle, for example, it can help to use two canes, one in either hand,
to provide leverage.

Physical therapists are also likely to make recommendations
to help improve walking and reduce the chance of falling. Below
are some suggestions you may hear from a therapist.

## Gait Improvement

When people who have Parkinson's disease walk, they have a tendency to take small, shuffling steps, and then have difficulty stopping. A strategy to avoid these problems is to think consciously about taking longer strides and about putting the entire foot down with each step. First the heel, then the toe. It can also be helpful to take frequent breaks during a walk. Resting seems to "reset" a more normal gait. When a person with Parkinson's disease stops, takes a short rest, and then resumes walking, the size of the initial steps often become quite normal.

Another trick for improving gait is to use visual cues to keep the size of each footstep regular. Place strips of masking tape on the floor, for example, at a comfortable distance apart for the person's age, weight, and sex; some people find that this strategy helps them walk with hardly a decrease in step size or speed!

Frozen gait can be another problem for people with Parkinson's disease. Frozen gait refers to an episode in which the feet seem to be stuck to the floor so that a person cannot move forward. This can be dangerous because it can happen suddenly and cause a fall, especially when someone is negotiating a curve. People who know they are prone to freezing episodes and falls sometimes use a cane or walker to keep themselves upright.

A freezing episode usually lasts just seconds or minutes. It is sometimes possible to move beyond the episode quickly and proceed even faster than before the freezing. People tend to discover their own ways of dealing with freezing episodes, but physical therapists also teach some useful and creative strategies. Here are a few:

- Visualize stepping over an imaginary target or line on the floor.

- Look ahead and focus on a distant point rather than on the floor directly underfoot.
- Count in a rhythmic cadence.
- March in place.

Many people find that one or all of these strategies can help restart the walking sequence.

The risk of freezing is related to medication schedules. Episodes of freezing tend to occur when medication is wearing off and the next dose is due. This emphasizes the importance of timing physical activity and medications in order to minimize the risk of injury. Time physical activity, as much as possible, to coincide with the first one to three hours after a dose of medication. As a general rule, a person with Parkinson's disease should pack up and take along at least one extra dose of medication whenever leaving the house. Many people also keep an extra dose of medication at work.

*Fall Prevention*

Fall prevention is one of the most important goals of physical therapy. More than 35 percent of people with advanced Parkinson's disease experience falls. Injuries tend to be minor cuts and bruises, but about 18 percent of falls result in the fracture of one or more bones.

Physical therapists teach multiple strategies to minimize the risk of falls, including the use of canes and walkers. To help a therapist design an individualized strategy for your family member, share details about the time and location of each fall. We recommend detailing falls and other events in a diary. Include information about activities leading up to the fall and the timing of medication in relation to the fall. This information is useful not only for the physical therapist but also for the neurologist.

The doctor can help by adjusting medication doses or their timing so that a patient is "on" during the most physically challenging periods of the day.

## Occupational Therapy

Occupational therapy (OT) is different from physical therapy and is a new concept for many people. Occupational therapy focuses on helping individuals maintain their function despite their limitations. OT addresses activities of daily living, such as bathing, dressing, shaving, applying make-up, eating, and writing. We tend to take these activities for granted until we can no longer perform them with our typical ease and speed.

Occupational therapists make recommendations for adaptive equipment and for establishing new routines that will allow for continued independence at home and work. One example of adaptive equipment is the long-handled shoehorn. This device is used to put shoes on without having to lean forward and run the risk of falling. Another example of adaptive equipment to minimize the risk of falls is a shower bench in the bathtub. To minimize tremor and ease the tension of eating, occupational therapists typically recommend using weighted eating utensils.

Micrographia, the small, cramped handwriting that is a symptom of Parkinson's disease, can be compensated for by the use of a computer. Typing on a keyboard can be much easier than writing with a pen or pencil. Occupational therapy treatments specific to those with Parkinson's disease include a home exercise program for the arms to maintain strength and promote flexibility, as well as the establishment of a routine for activities of daily living (bathing, dressing, applying make-up) that includes rest periods to compensate for fatigue.

There is some obvious expense to making life more comfortable for a person with a chronic condition like Parkinson's disease. Adapting the home to the patient's new reality can be an emotional and financial strain. But all parties—both the patients and their loved ones—must bear in mind that guilt and stress can only make the situation worse. Acknowledging from the start that this is a difficult adjustment period for everyone can help ease the tension.

## How Occupational and Physical Therapy Helps

So what do physical and occupational therapy sessions really do for people with Parkinson's disease? Let's look at a typical day in the life of a person with Parkinson's disease. We highlight activities that have been or can be improved with physical and occupational therapy.

*James is a fifty-six-year-old stockbroker who lives in Connecticut and works in New York City. James lives alone. He was diagnosed with Parkinson's disease six years ago, at which time he was experiencing an intermittent tremor in his right hand. He takes a dopamine agonist, ropinerole (Requip), and carbidopa/levodopa (Sinemet) four times a day. (Medications will be discussed later in this chapter.) James typically wakes up at 5:30 A.M. Thanks to a nightlight in his bedroom he does not have difficulty seeing at this early hour.*

*The medication James takes at bedtime works through the night, so he is only a little stiff and slow in the morning. Once he has turned off his alarm, James starts going over in his mind the movements he must perform in order to get out of bed without falling or feeling light-headed. Then he sits up, swings his legs over the side of the bed, and begins counting to fifteen. With that, he puts his feet down and, using his arms, pushes himself up into a standing position. As he walks across the bedroom to the bathroom, James visualizes each step he takes and also reminds himself to place first his heel firmly on the floor, followed by the ball of his foot, and finally by his toes.*

*Once in the bathroom, James has no difficulty using the toilet and taking a shower, thanks to assistive devices that were installed last year. James had noticed that he was having difficulty getting up from the toilet, so at the suggestion of his physical therapist, he installed a raised toilet seat with armrests. He also had a grab bar installed in the shower and always places a nonslip bath mat on the tub floor.*

*Although James has never slipped in the shower, a fall his seventy-nine-year-old mother had several years earlier, which resulted in a broken hip, made him acutely aware of the risks of not having adequate safety equipment in the bathroom. Very importantly, he does not rely on a towel bar to hold him up should he slip in the shower. A towel bar is designed to be strong enough to hold only the weight of a few towels. The grab bar James installed is textured, drilled securely into the wall studs, and designed specifically to help keep people upright should they need it. Now bathed and dressed, James heads to the kitchen for a full breakfast and his morning dose of medication.*

*Because James has difficulty with fine motor movement, he uses a rocker knife and other adaptive kitchen utensils to prepare and eat a meal of turkey sausage, egg-white omelet, and coffee. James learned about and ordered this equipment with the assistance of his occupational therapist. Since he was first diagnosed with Parkinson's disease, James has worked with his occupational therapist for three to four sessions every eighteen months.*

*After breakfast, James drives to the train station and manages, most mornings, to catch the 6:50 A.M. train to Manhattan. James and his neurologist have timed his morning medication dose so that it kicks in as his train reaches his destination, Grand Central Station. James gets off the train and walks to work without difficulty but remembers to place first his entire heel and then the ball and toes of his feet down. James tried using a cane six months ago after suffering a bout of the flu that left him feeling under the weather for several weeks, but he found that after a series of physical therapy ses-*

*sions focused on walking, he was able to return to his normal walking routine. James makes it to the office in time for the opening bell of the stock market and finds that the day flies by.*

*By the end of the work day, James is exhausted. His tremor is more pronounced and his ability to use a computer keyboard has markedly declined compared with the morning. Fortunately, James has a large, private office with a couch, so he takes a forty-five-minute nap before heading home. Prior to the nap, he takes a dose of medication so that he will be as mobile as possible for the walk back to the train station. On that walk, James focuses on taking big steps and on swinging his arms fully so that his gait is as normal and fast as possible. On most evenings he is home by 7 P.M.*

*James relaxes at home by preparing dinner and reading before he goes to bed. To help improve his mobility in bed, James uses satin sheets and an electric blanket. He stays warm and can also roll over in bed without being impeded by heavy blankets and linens.*

James is an example of someone who is aggressive in the treatment of his symptoms of Parkinson's disease. He maintains an active and independent lifestyle. Below is the story of Ellen, a woman who is less aggressive in her philosophy about illness and more sedentary than James. Nevertheless, Ellen obtained relief from some of her Parkinson symptoms by using multiple types of treatment.

*Ellen is seventy-four and was diagnosed with Parkinson's disease four years ago. She has been on the same medication regimen since she was first diagnosed and has not been very interested in learning about the disease or discussing her symptoms with her primary physician. Her daughter Nancy, by contrast, is frequently on the Internet searching for the latest information.*

*Nancy has noticed that her mother is slower in her movements and that her voice is more breathy. Nancy has also witnessed a few near-falls or trips that have gotten her worried about the possibility* that her mom could fall and break a bone. It was Nancy who made an appointment for her mom with Dr. Chen, a physician at the Parkinson's disease clinic at a nearby medical center.

Nancy accompanied her mom to the appointment and told the neurologist about the changes she had noticed in her mother's mobility and overall health. On the basis of the information provided by Ellen and Nancy and the exam itself, Dr. Chen changed Ellen's medication regimen.

Dr. Chen also arranged for PT sessions with a therapist who works extensively with people who have Parkinson's disease. The therapist focused on improving Ellen's gait and mobility. They worked together three times a week for eight weeks. In addition, Dr. Chen had the local visiting nurses association (VNA) assess Ellen in her home to ensure that she was safe and to determine if grab bars should be put in the tub or area rugs removed. Thus, by optimizing medications and taking advantage of the services provided by a multidisciplinary treatment team, Ellen improved her mobility and Nancy was reassured that her mom was able to continue to live independently.

## Speech Therapy

Speech-language therapists work with people who have a variety of disorders that affect the ability to make speech sounds clearly or at all. This includes people with speech rhythm and fluency problems and also those with voice-quality problems such as low pitch. Therapists concentrate on the mechanics of speaking, such as the movement of a person's tongue, lips, cheeks, throat, and upper-body muscles. Speech therapists also focus on aspects of breathing that are important for creating clear speech. They work with people who have difficulty eating and swallowing because of problems with the movement of their mouths. Some of these problems can appear in Parkinson's disease.

One such example is hypophonia, which refers to a reduction

in the loudness of the voice, as well as slowness in the rate of speaking. Friends and family often find that their loved one becomes difficult to understand because of hypophonia. Speech therapy can help patients make improvements in the intelligibility and loudness of their speech and their rate of speaking.

*Helena was first diagnosed with Parkinson's disease at the age of fifty-nine. At that time, she complained of a tremor in her right arm that she noticed every evening when she sat down to watch television. She was also bothered by a constant ache in her right arm. Helena's neurologist began treatment with a dopamine agonist, and both the severity of the tremor and the muscle soreness decreased significantly.*

*Shortly afterward, Helena's son, who was away at college, began to complain that it was hard to understand his mother on the telephone. Helena kept telling him that it was because the music he was playing in the background was too loud. Over the next two years, Helena's friends also began to tell her to speak up on the telephone, because they had trouble understanding her. At first, she ascribed the problem to old age and told her friends that they were becoming deaf. Eventually, however, she realized that even younger people had trouble understanding her. The next time Helena saw her neurologist, she learned that hypophonia is a symptom of Parkinson's disease. Her neurologist recommended speech therapy.*

*At the speech therapy sessions, Helena concentrated on speaking louder. For a month she worked with a speech therapist who had experience with speech disorders resulting from a range of physical conditions. Helena's friends and son began to comment that they had an easier time understanding her after she underwent speech therapy. She was able to make reservations at restaurants and book plane tickets over the telephone without any difficulty.*

Speech therapy first focuses on maneuvers to improve a person's natural vocal apparatus and then uses such things as amplification systems to augment the voice. A program called the Lee Silverman Voice Treatment (LSVT) program has been shown to be effective in improving both the volume and the speech of patients with Parkinson's disease.

The LSVT program is a compensatory maneuver that helps patients learn to speak in a louder voice. This is achieved by an intensive schedule of sixteen individual speech sessions over a one-month period. The program works to optimize sounds low in the throat. Studies have shown that 90 percent of patients improve after LSVT and that, of these, 80 percent maintain improvement in their voices for six to twelve months. The goal of speech therapy in Parkinson's disease is to improve and stabilize voice quality for a period of time. Speech therapy is not a one-time treatment; most people find that repeated therapy over the years helps to improve the quality of their voices.

It is important to remember that the more successful the drug therapy for Parkinson's disease, the greater the benefit from sessions with a speech therapist. Be sure to work closely with a neurologist to optimize medication regimens.

For people who find it difficult to maintain an adequate level of loudness in their voice, a repeat evaluation by a speech therapist can be very useful. A speech therapist can help improve communication by recommending aids like an easy-to-use message board or a voice amplification system. (See Figure 8.) Voice amplification systems consist of a lightweight speaker that is attached at the waist with a belt and equipped with a microphone. Patients who are being treated with deep-brain stimulation must be careful that the amplification product they select does not interfere with the functioning of the brain stimulator. It is important for these patients to be evaluated and treated by a speech therapist who has experience working with people with Parkinson's disease.

Hypophonia usually goes hand-in-hand with another condition called dysphagia. Dysphagia refers to difficulty swallowing,

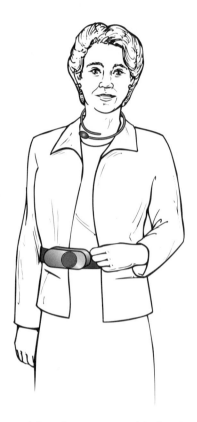

FIGURE 8.    Voice amplifier. The woman in this drawing is wearing a typical voice amplification system, consisting of a speaker that is worn discreetly around the waist and a microphone that rests gently around the neck. This system leaves the hands free and is light-weight.

and its severity is usually proportional to the decline in loudness of speech. A speech therapist can evaluate swallowing and recommend exercises and techniques for treating dysphagia. You should be aware that people with dysphagia have an increased risk of aspirating food. This means that instead of traveling down the esophagus to the stomach, food passes into the trachea and lungs. We have all had this experience, when food or drink goes down the wrong "pipe." In a person with Parkinson's disease, it is more difficult to cough up the aspirate, and they are thus at risk of developing pneumonia. Specific techniques taught by trained speech therapists can decrease the risk of aspiration.

## Medical Treatment

Medical treatment refers primarily to the use of medicines to relieve symptoms. To date, there are no medications to stop the progression of Parkinson's disease. The majority of patients use a single medication or combination of medications to relieve their symptoms. There are a variety of medications available to treat the symptoms of Parkinson's disease.

The decision about when to start taking medication is individual and based on a patient's degree of disability and discomfort. Everyone's comfort level will be different, of course, so when prescribing medications, doctors consider not only symptoms, but also the individuals' response to various dosages, and a host of social, occupational, and psychological issues.

From a doctor's perspective, the goal of pharmacological treatment is to help the patient function independently for as long as possible. Six classes of drugs are available to help accomplish that goal:

- anticholinergic agents
- antiviral drugs
- dopamine replacement agents
- dopamine agonists
- inhibitors of the enzyme monoamine oxidase B (MAO-B)
- inhibitors of the enzyme catechol-o-methyl transferase (COMT)

*Table 2*   Medications used in the treatment of Parkinson's disease

| Drug class | Generic name | Brand name |
| --- | --- | --- |
| Anticholinergic | Benztropine<br>Trihexyphenidyl | Cogentin<br>Artane |
| Antiviral | Amantadine | Symmetrel |
| Dopamine agonists | Bromocriptine<br>Pergolide<br>Ropinerole<br>Pramipexole | Parlodel<br>Permax<br>Requip<br>Mirapex |
| Dopamine replacement | Carbidopa/levodopa | Sinemet |
| COMT inhibitor | Entacapone<br>Tolcapone | Comtan<br>Tasmar |
| MAO-B inhibitor | Selegiline | Deprenyl |
| Combination dopamine replacement + COMT inhibitor | Carbidopa/levodopa + entacapone | Stalevo |

Each medication has a generic name, which is listed first in this book, and a brand name, which is listed in parentheses after the generic name. (See Table 2.)

So what is the difference between a brand-name drug and its generic counterpart? When a pharmaceutical company develops a new drug, the company applies to a government patent office for a patent. This patent gives the company the right to sell its drug without competition. In most countries the life of a patent is twenty years from registration. The purpose of a patent is to allow a company to recoup its investment and make a profit. At the same time, the company applies to the national trademark office to obtain permission for the exclusive use of a particular name. This name is the brand name of the particular drug. After a review, the brand name is registered to the company and then becomes the property of that company. After a patent expires, other pharmaceutical companies may manufacture and sell the original drug as a generic drug. The generic drug must contain the same medicinal ingredient(s) as the brand-name version. Since less time is needed to do the initial research, generic drugs typically cost less than their brand-name counterparts.

## Anticholinergic Agents

Anticholinergic agents are the oldest class of medications used for Parkinson's disease. They work by blocking the effects of a neurotransmitter called acetylcholine and are most effective in reducing rest tremor and rigidity. However, they have side effects that typically limit their use. The side effects include dry mouth, constipation, urinary retention, blurred vision, confusion, and difficulty with concentration.

## Antiviral Agents

Amantadine (brand name Symmetrel) is also used to treat Parkinson's disease. Amantadine is classified as an antiviral drug. We do not fully understand how it works in Parkinson's disease. It is thought to work by augmenting the release of dopamine from those neurons that are viable and producing dopamine. Amantadine produces limited improvement in bradykinesia (slow movement), rigidity, and rest tremor. Amantadine is helpful in controlling dyskinesias that can develop later in the course of Parkinson's disease. (Dyskinesias are discussed in greater detail in Chapter 5.) Possible side effects include lower-extremity edema (swelling caused by accumulation of fluid), confusion, and hallucinations.

## Dopamine Replacement

Dopamine replacement is the cornerstone of therapy for Parkinson's disease. (Recall that Parkinson's disease results from the loss of brain cells that produce dopamine.) Patients actually take a drug called levodopa rather than dopamine. Levodopa is a natural precursor to dopamine and is given in combination with another medication called carbidopa. Carbidopa helps the levodopa enter the brain by blocking the breakdown of the drug in the bloodstream before it enters the brain itself.

Levodopa is most effective in reducing tremor, rigidity, and akinesia. The most common side effects, seen with the onset of treatment, are nausea and abdominal cramping. Long-term treatment with levodopa or the dopamine agonists (discussed below) is associated with two potential types of complications: hourly fluctuations in motor state and dyskinesias. It is not clear if these complications are due to the medications, the progression of the underlying disease, or some complex interaction between these two factors. The long-term complications are discussed in greater detail in Chapter 5.

### Dopamine Agonists

Dopamine agonists for Parkinson's disease work by directly stimulating dopamine receptors on brain cells. An agonist is a drug that binds to and activates a receptor on a cell, leading to changes within that cell. Dopamine agonists fool the brain into thinking that there is more dopamine present than is actually the case. There are several different dopamine agonists, and they can be used alone or in combination with levodopa therapy. (See Figure 9.)

The older dopamine agonists, bromocriptine (Parlodel) and pergolide (Permax), are less specific in their actions than the newer agents. The newer dopamine agonists, pramipexole (Mirapex) and ropinerole (Requip), are thus, in theory, less likely to cause unpleasant side effects. However, the theoretical benefit to the newer dopamine agonists has not been conclusively demonstrated in long-term clinical trials. Compared with levodopa,

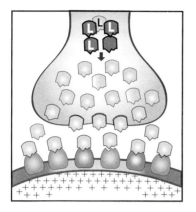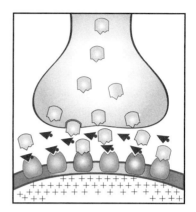

FIGURE 9.    Action of levodopa and dopamine receptor agonists. Left panel: Levodopa (L) is taken up by brain cells and converted to dopamine. A mixture of the small amount of dopamine that the brain cell made on its own and the dopamine resulting from the ingestion of levodopa medication is then released and binds to receptors on the next brain cell.

Right panel: Dopamine agonists enter the brain and bind directly to dopamine receptors because they have a chemical structure similar to that of dopamine. After transmitting information by binding to the receptors, the dopamine agonists are then released from the receptor (represented by the black arrows) and broken down into inactive components.

both the new and the old dopamine agonists cause a lower occurrence of dyskinesias and a higher occurrence of confusion and hallucinations. To minimize the risk of intolerable side effects, patients should start with a small dose of medication and then slowly increase the total daily dosage.

## MAO-B Inhibitors of Dopamine Metabolism

Inhibitors of dopamine metabolism are also used to treat Parkinson's disease. Metabolism refers to the breakdown of a particular medication. Thus, agents that inhibit the metabolism of dopamine will allow the dopamine to remain in its active state for a longer period. Selegiline (Deprenyl) is an inhibitor of dopamine metabolism. It inhibits the enzyme monoamine oxidase B (MAO-B), which acts in the central nervous system by breaking down dopamine. Common side effects include dry mouth and dizziness.

## COMT Inhibitors of Dopamine Metabolism

Entacapone (Comtan) is another inhibitor of dopamine metabolism. Entacapone inhibits the activity of the enzyme called catechol-o-methyl transferase (COMT), which breaks down levodopa. Entacapone is taken in conjunction with a tablet of carbidopa/levodopa and acts to increase the amount of levodopa that reaches the brain. Common side effects include abdominal pain and fatigue. The benefits of entacapone treatment include a reduction in total daily levodopa dose and an improvement in the length of time of optimal mobility. (See Figure 10.)

Recently a new combination pill of entacapone with carbidopa and levodopa has become available. The brand name of this drug is Stalevo. The advantage to this combination medication is that it reduces the number of tablets a person has to take on a daily basis. Common side effects of Stalevo include nausea and headache.

Tolcapone (Tasmar) is another inhibitor of catechol-o-methyl transferase. Like entacapone, tolcapone is taken in conjunction with a tablet of carbidopa/levodopa and acts to increase the amount of levodopa that reaches the brain. A rare but fatal risk from taking tolcapone is acute liver failure. Because of this risk, the use of tolcapone is typically limited to people who either cannot tolerate or do not derive benefits from other medications for their Parkinson's disease.

Below are some commonly asked questions about medications used to treat Parkinson's disease.

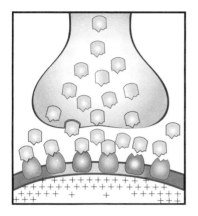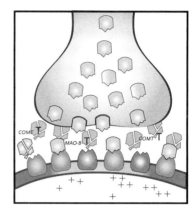

FIGURE 10. The metabolism of dopamine in the brain. Two enzymes, COMT and MAO-B, are present in the space between two nerve cells. These enzymes work separately to break down dopamine.

### ARE THERE POSSIBLE INTERACTIONS BETWEEN PARKINSON'S DISEASE MEDICATIONS AND OVER-THE-COUNTER (OTC) DRUGS?

Yes, there may be interactions, depending on the specific combination of Parkinson's medication and nonprescription drugs. Check with your doctor before taking any over-the-counter medications. In fact, you should ask about drug interactions with the start of any new prescription or OTC medicine.

### WHAT SHOULD BE DONE ABOUT A FORGOTTEN DOSE OF MEDICATION?

Here is the general rule: The dose should be taken if it is remembered within an hour of when it was due. Otherwise, it should be skipped and taken at the next scheduled time. It is important that doses *not* be doubled up.

### HOW CRITICAL IS IT THAT MEDICATIONS BE TAKEN AT A PARTICULAR TIME?

There are several reasons for maintaining a daily schedule of medication doses. First, establishing a schedule makes it less likely that medications will be forgotten. Second, maintaining relatively steady levels of medication in the bloodstream (and, therefore, in the brain), allows a patient to control his or her symptoms to the greatest extent possible. Third, spacing out the medication doses at fairly regular intervals makes it less likely that side effects such as abdominal cramps or nausea will occur; these side effects are more common when there are excessively high levels of medication in the bloodstream.

### SHOULD MEDICATION BE TAKEN BEFORE OR AFTER MEALS?

The timing of doses depends on the medication. Carbidopa/ levodopa (Sinemet), for example, is best taken on an empty stomach at least thirty minutes before a meal or one hour afterward. Some of the dopamine agonists, such as pramipexole (Mirapex) and ropinerole (Requip), by contrast, can cause nausea if taken on an empty stomach. It is best to review these issues with both a doctor and a pharmacist, to be certain that the instructions are clear and well understood.

### HOW DOES TRAVELING TO A DIFFERENT TIME ZONE AFFECT MEDICATION SCHEDULES?

Medications are meant to help a patient with Parkinson's disease move more easily and quickly. Because the drugs used for PD alleviate symptoms and have no effect on the overall course of the disease, it is okay to make adjustments to the medication schedule if traveling to a different time zone.

Here is an example that Dr. Sharma uses for her patients: Let's say, for example, that you live in New York and fly to London. A typical flight leaves New York at 6:30 P.M. and reaches London at 6:30 A.M., local time, which is 1:30 in the morning to your body. On the day of the trip, and while in the plane, you should continue to take your medication according to New York time. The issue becomes what to do in the hour before the plane lands, because you want to be able to move quickly and easily once you disembark from the plane. You could take a tablet of carbidopa/levodopa (Sinemet) forty-five minutes before the plane lands. This is about the time the flight attendants announce that the plane has begun its descent. This pill will kick in just after the plane has landed, when you will need to move around the cabin, pick up your belongings, and disembark. Remember that taking an additional pill will not have any long-term effect on the course of the Parkinson's disease. After you disembark, pass through customs, and finally reach your hotel, you will undoubtedly be exhausted and ready for a nap. After the nap, it will be late morning or early afternoon in London. At this time, you can resume your usual medication regimen on the basis of local time.

### WHAT HAPPENS IF MEDICATIONS RUN OUT WHILE WE'RE IN ANOTHER COUNTRY?

Because the laws regulating availability of medication vary widely from country to country, you should always take along an ample supply. At least two weeks before the trip check the number of pills on hand. Call the pharmacy to get an additional refill, if needed. This will give you enough time to get the additional medication if the doctor has to write a new prescription.

## Surgical Treatment

Although many medications are available for treating early and moderately advanced Parkinson's disease, their use is limited in more advanced cases. This is where surgery can be useful. Several surgical procedures are either currently available or being actively studied in research laboratories. Information about them will continue to grow in the next several years.

Surgical approaches to treating advanced Parkinson's disease fall into one of three categories:

- restorative (cell transplantation or the use of brain cell growth factors)
- ablative (thalamotomy or pallidotomy)
- electrophysiological (deep-brain stimulation, or DBS)

### Restorative Surgery

Cell transplantation is still an experimental approach to the treatment of Parkinson's disease. The goal is to replace the lost dopamine-producing brain neurons. At this time, four different sources of dopamine-producing cells are being studied.

*Human fetal neuronal cells.* In animal models of Parkinson's disease, transplants of fetal tissue have been shown to work reasonably well. The outcome in humans, however, is not so encouraging. In a recent study in which human embryonic dopamine neurons were transplanted into the brains of patients with severe Parkinson's disease, there was no significant, long-term improvement in symptoms.

*Human adult precursor cells.* We don't yet know if cells that have the capability to transform into neurons exist in the adult human brain. If they do, it may be possible to isolate them in the laboratory and coax them into becoming dopamine-producing neurons, which could then be surgically implanted into the human brain.

Previous studies in patients with Parkinson's disease used cells not from the brain but from the adult adrenal gland. The adrenal gland is a tiny conglomeration of cells that sits atop the kidney. Some cells within the adrenal gland produce dopamine. The adrenal dopamine cells were isolated and then inserted into the brain of some patients with Parkinson's disease. Unfortunately, the results were disappointing.

*Embryonic stem cells.* Embryonic stem (ES) cells are initially obtained from a developing human embryo about four to seven days after an egg is fertilized. ES cells are pluripotent, meaning that they can develop into any number of the specialized cells of the human body. Once removed, the ES cells are grown in the laboratory, where they increase in number and can be induced to change their characteristics.

The thought is that ES cells can be used to treat a variety of diseases, including Parkinson's disease, Alzheimer's disease, and diabetes. Even with increased funding to accelerate the rate of research, there is considerable work to be done before ES cell–based therapies are ready to be used in humans, even experimentally.

For Parkinson's disease, researchers hope to stimulate ES cells into becoming dopamine-producing cells that could then be transplanted into the human brain. The ES cells would provide an unlimited supply of the highly specialized, dopamine-producing neurons. However, the secrets of how to change embryonic stem cells into dopamine-producing neurons and then to insert them safely among other brain cells have yet to be discovered.

*Xenotransplantation.* Xenotransplantation refers to the transfer of nonhuman tissue into the human body. The procedure carries the risk of introducing animal viruses or bacteria into humans. A recent study evaluated the safety and efficacy of a procedure to transplant embryonic brain cells from pigs into twelve people with Parkinson's disease. One year after the surgery, there was no evidence of infection by a pig virus in the recipients. However, there was no significant improvement in the UPDRS score, either. These results indicate that xenotransplantation may be safe in humans, but its benefits remain uncertain. Research to refine the techniques used in xenotransplantation, with an emphasis on minimizing the risk of introducing animal viruses into humans, continues.

An alternative approach to xenotransplantation is to deliver growth factors to the brain that would promote the development and survival of dopamine-producing neurons. One of the compounds under study is called glial-cell–derived neurotrophic factor (GDNF). In a recent study, five people with Parkinson's disease underwent surgical implantation of a pump device for delivering the GDNF. The pump portion was placed in the abdomen and connected by thin plastic tubing to the basal ganglia of the brain. (Abdominal placement makes the pump easily accessible to physicians.)

GDNF was put in the pump, which then delivered the compound to the dopamine-producing neurons of the basal ganglia. The results of this small study indicate that this method is safe for delivering GDNF to the brain, and may also be helpful for improving the motor symptoms of Parkinson's disease. However, a study of only five people is not large enough for reaching definitive conclusions. A larger study is currently being conducted to determine if GDNF, delivered directly to the basal ganglia, will be beneficial for people with Parkinson's disease.

### Ablative Surgery

Ablative surgery is a technique that was introduced before oral medications were available for treating Parkinson's disease. It is used to destroy specific structures of the brain within the basal ganglia where the symptoms of PD arise. One of two distinct regions of the basal ganglia are targeted for destruction, depending on a patient's symptoms. The surgery creates damage that is irreversible.

*Pallidotomy.* Some patients whose symptoms do not respond to medication can still benefit from ablative surgery. In a surgical procedure called a pallidotomy, a surgeon creates a lesion in a portion of the brain called the globus pallidus. This procedure is recommended for some patients who experience bradykinesia, rigidity, tremor, and significant drug-induced dyskinesia despite optimal medical therapy.

*Thalamotomy.* In another surgical treatment, called a thalamotomy, a neurosurgeon makes a lesion in a region of the brain's thalamus. Thalamotomy is recommended for those with Parkinson's disease who have an asymmetric, severe, and medically intractable tremor.

## Electrophysiological Treatment

In deep-brain stimulation (DBS), high-frequency electrical pulses are applied via a wire or wires to one of several locations in the basal ganglia. (See Figure 11.) DBS requires a surgical procedure in which a device for providing electrical stimulation (like a pacemaker) is placed under the skin of the chest. The wires attached to the device are threaded into the subthalamic nucleus, thalamus, or globus pallidus of the brain. The electrical stimulation is thought to block the signals that cause the disabling motor symptoms in Parkinson's disease. The extent of stimulation can be adjusted by an experienced movement disorder neurologist using a hand-held device that is placed on the surface of the skin, just above the site where the device was placed (typically just below the collarbone).

DBS surgery is a major undertaking and requires an extensive evaluation at a Parkinson's disease center as well as thoughtful consideration by the patient, patient's partner, and family members. It is important to weigh the risk and benefits of the surgery carefully.

Below are some frequently asked questions about surgery.

### DO I HAVE TO SHAVE MY HEAD PRIOR TO SURGERY?

The area around the region where the surgeon will operate has to be shaved. Many people opt to shave their entire head, so that the hair can then grow back uniformly.

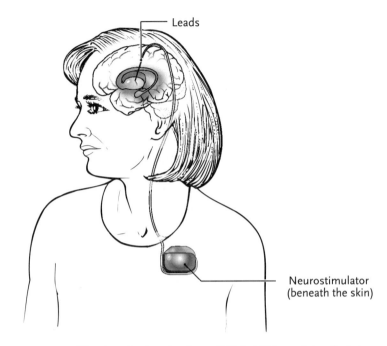

Leads

Neurostimulator
(beneath the skin)

FIGURE 11.    The deep-brain stimulator (DBS). DBS consists of a battery source that rests below the collarbone and just under the skin.
Electrodes from the battery are threaded into the brain, where they
generate a magnetic field whose size can be adjusted by changing the
settings on the battery. A neurologist can make these changes during
an office visit by using a hand-held device that is placed on top of the
battery. Adjustments to the DBS are non-invasive.

### WILL I FEEL PAIN DURING THE SURGERY?

Patients are given a local anesthetic so they won't feel any pain
when the hard, bony skull is cut. However, because some patient
cooperation is required during the procedure, the patient is
often awake. If you're considering this surgery, discuss anesthesia
options with your surgeon and anesthesiologist before the day of
surgery.

## WILL I FEEL PAIN AFTER THE SURGERY?

As the connective tissue, muscle, and skin heal at the incision site, you may feel some discomfort or sharp pain. This is part of the normal healing process. The pain will subside as the tissues heal.

## DO I HAVE TO BE CAREFUL AROUND ELECTRONIC DEVICES AFTER DBS SURGERY?

Most electrical appliances used at home and equipment used at work do not interfere with the DBS device. This includes microwave ovens, computers, and cell phones. However, large stereo speakers have magnets that might turn off the DBS device. Also, patients should be careful about approaching and going through airport or store security portals. These portals may have enough electromagnetic energy to cause an increase in the amount of stimulation given off by the DBS device. Should you undergo surgery and have a DBS device implanted, you will receive detailed information about this and other safety concerns. You will also receive an identification card to carry with you at all times.

After the patient has recovered from surgery, the stimulator is turned on by means of a device that is held up to the chest. The advantage of DBS is that once the unit is in place, the degree of electrical stimulation can be easily adjusted through the controller. With thalamotomy and pallidotomy, in contrast, the lesion is fixed and permanent.

Surgical treatment for medication-resistant Parkinson's disease is an important and rapidly expanding therapeutic option. In carefully selected cases, surgical treatment can have a very positive effect on symptoms. It is crucial that anyone considering surgery be evaluated and screened at a center that specializes in surgical treatments of Parkinson's disease.

Information about treatments for Parkinson's disease, from physical therapy through brain surgery, is complex and may seem overwhelming. Bear in mind that each patient is unique; while one drug or procedure may work well for one person, it may not be appropriate for someone else. The key to understanding your situation is to ask questions until you have an explanation that makes you feel satisfied. By seeking as much information as possible about your condition or that of someone you love, you will be able to make intelligent decisions.

# 5

# Treatment Challenges and Setbacks

*Roy's wife of thirty-five years, Darlene, had been taking carbidopa/ levodopa (Sinemet) for her Parkinson's disease for four years. At the time of Darlene's diagnosis, she had a resting tremor that was quite noticeable and a walking speed that was about half of what it had been. (She was taking two times longer than Roy to walk a city block.) With medication, Darlene had been doing quite well. She was taking Sinemet three times a day, which left the tremor barely noticeable unless she was anxious or upset. Roy had remarked to the doctor that, with Darlene on medication, their walking pace was still slow but had increased by about 30 percent.*

*In the past six months, however, Roy and Darlene both realized that a change was taking place and suspected that the Sinemet might be losing its effectiveness. Darlene was taking the medication at 7:00 in the morning, 5:00 in the afternoon, and 11:00 at night.*

*Gradually, Darlene realized that she was stiffer and slower than usual when she woke in the morning. Instead of getting dressed and preparing breakfast for her husband and herself in a total of forty-five minutes, she needed the whole time just to get dressed. Roy had started making their breakfast.*

*In addition, they were missing their usual 3:00 walk because Darlene was weak and stiff again in the late afternoon. She wanted to sit instead of walk. Roy noticed that her forearm tremor increased around that time and that, because of a continuous shaking, Darlene was complaining of soreness by 7:00 or 8:00 each evening.*

*Roy became concerned that in another few months Darlene
would not be able to go for their daily walks at all. He worried that
she would end up in a wheelchair and that he would not be able to
take care of her at home. Roy began having difficulty sleeping at
night, but he did not discuss his fears with Darlene out of concern
that she would become scared, too. A visit to their neurologist confirmed that Darlene's medication was less effective than it had been.
The doctor recommended that Darlene try a new medication
regimen.*

This reduction in the duration of relief from a drug treatment
is known as the wearing-off effect. In the early stage of Parkinson's disease, which can last for many years, an individual
usually takes medication three times a day and may even occasionally forget to take a dose without feeling any worsening of
symptoms. As the disease progresses, however, some people begin to experience a wearing-off of their medication.

At first, the person who used to forget to take an occasional
dose begins to take the medication precisely at the prescribed
times because he or she can sense that the stiffness or tremor is
returning. Now the patient takes a new dose of medication not
according to the clock, but rather according to the onset of symptoms. As a partner or close friend or family member, you may
notice, in the hour before a dose of medication is due, that walking pace and speaking have slowed down.

Sometimes the wearing-off effect can be even more pronounced, especially in people who do not exhibit any signs of
Parkinson's disease when their medication is working. After
four or five hours without taking a dose of medication, they suddenly become stiff, slow, and unable to walk without risking a
fall. In an "off" state, it is also common for people to feel anxious and be slower in processing information and responding to
questions. It is not that they do not understand what is being

asked or what is going on around them; it is just that the brain, like the body, is working slowly.

The reason for the wearing-off effect is unknown. It may be related to the progression of the disease. It may be that patients stop responding as well to the drug; in other words, they develop a tolerance. Another theory is that additional dopamine-producing neurons in the brain have died so that as the medication wears off, there is even less natural dopamine left in the brain to exert a continued effect. Researchers are testing these different hypotheses. Most likely, the variations in response to levodopa treatment over time are the result of a complex imbalance between the imperfect addition of dopamine in the form of oral medication, and the ongoing loss of dopamine-producing nerve cells in the brain.

An early sign of the wearing-off effect to be aware of is when improvement from a dose of carbidopa/levodopa is followed by a relatively rapid recurrence of symptoms. For example, a rest tremor that used to be controlled for eight hours after a dose of medicine may begin to recur after only six hours. Initially, the wearing-off effect will be predictable. This makes it possible to schedule activities that require fine motor control, like dressing and eating, in the two to three hours immediately after a dose of medication.

The wearing-off effect can be minimized. One approach is to use a longer-acting form of carbidopa/levodopa, known as Sinemet CR. The CR stands for controlled release. The difference between a tablet of regular carbidopa/levodopa and a CR tablet is that the regular tablet is fully absorbed within one hour of ingestion, whereas the CR tablet takes longer, approximately two hours, to be fully absorbed. Another approach is to add a second drug, entacapone (Comtan), which prolongs the life of levodopa in the brain. Yet another choice is to increase the frequency of carbidopa/levodopa doses. For example, a person might take carbidopa/levodopa every three or four hours rather than every six to eight hours.

Many people who experience wearing-off effects learn to schedule their activities so that they are at home, or seated comfortably at work, when the medication is due to wear off. They also get into the habit of keeping an extra set of pills near the chair where they typically sit, along with a glass of water, so that they will not have to struggle to get up and walk as the medication wears off. The added anxiety of having to rush to get medication can make it even more difficult to move quickly. Remarkably, once the next dose of medication kicks in and someone is "on," movements are quite smooth and easy to initiate. It is not unusual for people to have essentially normal, or almost normal, neurological exams when they are "on."

## Other Motor Complications

People who have been treated for Parkinson's disease for many years may experience other motor complications in addition to wearing-off effects:

- Slowness or tremor at a time of the day different from the usual early morning occurrence, for example.
- Muscle contraction (dystonia), particularly in the feet, neck, and trunk. These contractions can be painful and protracted. Dystonia tends to occur when plasma levels of levodopa rise or fall. The most common form of dystonia consists of morning or evening foot cramps.
- Repetitive, uncontrolled movements (dyskinesia) involving the arms, legs, trunk, or head. Dyskinesias usually occur when blood levels of levodopa are at their peak and can involve rapid movement of arms, legs, or portions of the head and neck. Unlike dystonia, which can be quite pain-

ful, dyskinesias are generally more emotionally upsetting than physically uncomfortable. Many people with Parkinson's disease would rather cope with uncontrolled movements than be unable to move at all, and so they opt to continue taking levodopa. Often those watching someone who is dyskinetic feel uncomfortable and have an urge to do something to stop the uncontrolled movements. It is important to keep in mind that a medication regimen is adjusted for the benefit of the individual with Parkinson's disease, not for those who live or work closely with that person. Later in this chapter we discuss strategies for minimizing dyskinesias.

- Motor fluctuations. Gradually, the periods when the medication is effective may become shorter and shorter. Motor fluctuations become common, and some people experience an on-off effect whereby they have rapidly alternating periods of dyskinesia (excessive motor activity) and immobility.

- Temporarily ineffective medications. Some people may occasionally find that a particular dose of medication is not effective at all. This is known as the skipped-dose phenomenon and typically occurs on a random basis. One method for minimizing the risk of experiencing a skipped dose phenomenon is to reduce the amount of protein in the diet. Protein in the stomach interferes with the absorption of levodopa. Thus, eating less protein may help to maximize the absorption of carbidopa/levodopa from the stomach into the bloodstream. Some people find that if they limit the amount of protein they eat at breakfast and lunch, their response to levodopa is maximized during the day. But bear in mind that no diet should be initiated without first consulting the treating physician. A significant risk of a low-protein diet is weight loss and malnutrition.

Remember that every person with Parkinson's disease experiences a unique combination of symptoms and responses to medication. It is important to work closely with a neurologist who is skilled in treating Parkinson's disease, in order to maximize your abilities or those of your loved one. If you live in an area where there are no neurologists nearby, your local physician can be an effective partner in your care by working with a neurologist whom you see once or twice a year.

Below are some commonly asked questions about motor problems associated with Parkinson's disease.

### CAN ANYTHING BE DONE TO AVOID DYSKINESIAS?

The way that dyskinesias develop is poorly understood. What is clear, however, is that the two main factors that contribute to the development of dyskinesias are levodopa and the severity of Parkinson's disease itself. The combination of these two factors appears to lead to changes in the brain that result in dyskinesias. On the basis of this limited understanding of how dyskinesias develop, clinicians have come up with several strategies to stave off the onset of dyskinesias.

One strategy is to delay the use of levodopa and then, once it is needed for control of the symptoms of Parkinson's disease, use as small a daily dose as possible.

Another method is to decrease the total daily amount of levodopa. Although less levodopa will help to minimize dyskinesias, it will also result in a recurrence of more symptoms of Parkinson's disease.

Yet another strategy is to even out the levodopa dose throughout the day, minimizing the number of peaks and valleys in brain dopamine concentration. Practically speaking, this means taking pills more frequently throughout the day. Although this can be inconvenient, it does help to maximize mobility throughout the day.

A fourth strategy for managing dyskinesias is to add the drug amantadine (Symmetrel) to the daily drug regimen. Amantadine was developed as an antiviral medication and is used to prevent and treat respiratory infections caused by the influenza A virus. It is also used to minimize dyskinesias in Parkinson's disease. We do not fully understand how amantadine works in the brain of someone with Parkinson's disease, though it is thought to promote the release of dopamine from those neurons that continue to produce it.

Despite concerns over the role of long-term levodopa use in the development of dyskinesias, it is important to remember that our understanding of dyskinesias is imperfect. Physicians treating Parkinson's disease do not recommend that patients hold off taking levodopa if they find that their Parkinson's symptoms make it difficult to participate in regular activities. The doctor's foremost goal in the treatment of Parkinson's disease is to keep the patient functioning independently and normally for as long as possible.

*I'VE HEARD ABOUT THE BENEFITS OF A LOW-PROTEIN DIET FOR PARKINSON'S PATIENTS. IS THIS A GOOD IDEA, AND DOES IT WORK FOR EVERYONE?*

For people who experience marked "on-off" symptoms, a low-protein diet in which the bulk of the daily protein requirement is eaten at dinner can be beneficial. By marked on-off we mean that before a dose of Sinemet a person is extremely rigid and then, thirty to forty-five minutes after taking it, becomes dyskinetic.

After we eat, protein from food is broken down by the stomach and small intestines, and then absorbed into the bloodstream. In someone with Parkinson's disease, the same absorption process is used to get carbidopa/levodopa into the bloodstream. Hence, when a person eats a lot of protein, its absorption can interfere with the absorption of carbidopa/ levodopa. Most people do not have marked fluctuations in response to carbidopa/levodopa, so interference from protein is not a significant problem. For people who experience marked "off" periods and dyskinesias, though, limiting protein intake at breakfast and lunch may improve the absorption of carbidopa/ levodopa and help maintain a steady level of the drug in the bloodstream.

*I'VE HEARD THAT A DRUG HOLIDAY CAN IMPROVE THE EFFECTIVENESS OF LEVODOPA. IS THIS A GOOD IDEA?*

A drug holiday refers to a period of time when a person stops taking his or her medication. Drug holidays have been evaluated as a way to reduce the risk of developing levodopa-associated dyskinesias. Although some people experience an improvement in dyskinesias when their levodopa treatment is reinstated following a drug holiday, the improvement does not last for longer than several weeks or months. For those with advanced Parkinson's disease, in whom a lack of treatment would result in significant immobility and the danger of falls, the risks of a drug holiday are significant and any benefit unproven. Because there is no clear-cut benefit to taking a drug holiday and because the risk of significant complications from enduring the symptoms of Parkinson's disease without treatment is significant, drug holidays are not recommended.

# 6

# Finding the Help You Need

There is no reason for Parkinson's patients and their families to go without information and emotional support that will help them manage the disease. Many resources are available.

Some families want information about the disease itself. Others want to know about medications, long-term care, or clinical research studies. Still others want to learn new skills for coping with the emotional aspects of living with a loved one who has a chronic disease. Whatever a family's question, there is an answer somewhere and an agency trying to make it easy to find.

We offer several case studies as examples of ways people find what they need and want. The first is about a young man named Ramon who was just about to launch a career ten years in the making when he learned of his mother's Parkinson's disease. He thought he might have to abandon his plans and move in with his parents.

*When Ramon completed graduate school in chemical engineering, he decided to move back to his home town to accept an exciting job at a local high-technology company. Ramon had left for college almost ten years earlier and had been home only for brief vacations. He and his parents agreed that he would move back into the family house for a short time to save money for a down payment on a place of his own. They all thought that a year would be a reasonable amount of time for him to work and save.*

*It wasn't long before Ramon noticed that something was not quite right with his mom, Gloria. She had always been extremely active around the house and community. Now he noticed that she stayed home a lot. Sometimes when they were sitting around her right arm would shake. It didn't take much urging for Ramon to convince Gloria to make an appointment to see her doctor. The doctor made a tentative diagnosis of Parkinson's disease and sent Gloria to a specialist for additional evaluation.*

*Ramon and his mom visited the specialist, a neurologist, together. When the doctor confirmed the diagnosis of Parkinson's disease, Ramon felt shocked and deeply dismayed. How could his mom, who took care of everything and was always busy, have a chronic illness? What would happen to her? And how could his dad, who had never done any housework, cope if he had to take care of his wife and their home? Ramon decided be would abandon his plans to move out. Instead he would stay to help his parents. He even considered quitting his job.*

*Gloria, by contrast, took the news in stride. She began using the medications the neurologist had prescribed and even attended several meetings of a support group for people with Parkinson's disease. After a while, however, she realized that she was not comfortable sharing her feelings in public, and she stopped going.*

*Gloria's husband, Eduardo, was perhaps the biggest problem of all. He refused to believe that anything was wrong and became upset if he even heard the words "Parkinson's disease."*

*Ramon spent hours on the Internet trying to learn all that he could about Parkinson's disease. He was encouraged to read that people with Parkinson's disease are able to live independently for many years. Ramon got involved with the National Parkinson Foundation (NPF), one of the many organizations that provide educational support for people with PD and their family members. After reading about Parkinson's disease and talking with members of the NPF, Ramon realized that his mom would probably do well for many years to come. The following spring, right on target, Ramon hired a realtor and began house hunting.*

The second case study is about a couple who needed some urging from the doctor to learn more about how to manage the behavior changes that sometimes emerge in families when Parkinson's disease is diagnosed.

*Dan and his wife, Marjorie, both retired in the same year from their jobs as school teachers. They had taught in the same district for thirty-five years. They had raised two children who were now adult and independent. The couple looked forward to a fun retirement together with time for exercise, travel, gardening, and their five grandchildren.*

*Evenings were for reading and watching television, something that they had not had time to do during the school year. Marjorie noticed that as they sat Dan had a tendency to shake his right leg. At first it looked like a nervous habit, but then she realized that his right arm was shaking, too. It was six months before Dan finally agreed to see the family doctor. Three months later, a neurologist at a movement disorder center confirmed a diagnosis of Parkinson's disease.*

*Dan and Marjorie were stunned by the news. They had anticipated an active retirement. Instead, Marjorie became very protective and would not let Dan leave the house without her. She began driving him everywhere, rather than let him drive alone, and urged him to "get his rest" by napping daily. She insisted on taking him to his barber and to the library, and she even pulled a chair alongside the indoor pool to watch him while he swam his laps. Dan, by contrast, began taking medication and found that the tremor improved significantly. Once he became used to taking medication regularly he felt like his usual self and told Marjorie that her concern was excessive and suffocating. When the doctor noticed the tension between the couple, he suggested ways they could better cope with Parkinson's disease.*

## Illness Is a Family Affair

A diagnosis of Parkinson's disease affects *all* family members, not just the person with the disease. It excludes no one. Parkinson's disease represents an emotional and physical challenge for everyone connected with the person diagnosed.

For adult children, the disease may be the first sign of the inevitable change in the parent-child relationship. The child, accustomed to being the one who is cared for, suddenly becomes the one who must provide support and be responsible.

Families with young children face a special challenge. Young children may not understand the disease but are quick to see that something is different, that Mom or Dad has tremors or difficulty walking. They may also have a hard time understanding the parent's softer speech. Kids need assurance that they are loved and safe. Even young children can benefit from some concrete information about the disease, for instance, the fact that Parkinson's disease is not contagious.

Bear in mind that teenagers may find it embarrassing to have a parent with Parkinson's disease. Some teens find it helpful to sort out their feelings through visits to a professional counselor. Others get satisfaction from helping with tasks that have been the sole responsibility of the parent with Parkinson's disease. Teenagers may also benefit from being told that they are not expected to act as caregivers, and that their plan to leave home and enter college or the working world will remain unchanged.

For the helping partner, a diagnosis of PD opens up a door to a completely new world, one that most people never imagined they would be entering and about which they know very little.

New kinds of choices confront the partner, including decisions about doctors, medications, care, health insurance, family economics, friendships, work, and so on. Sex can also become a significant issue between couples when one partner has Parkinson's disease. As odd as it may seem at first, coping successfully with chronic illness can have the unexpected effect of bringing a family closer together. By adapting to a new situation, people often find themselves feeling stronger, better adjusted, and more satisfied with themselves and their relationships.

## Sources of Help

There are many sources of information for people affected by Parkinson's disease. In fact, there is more than you ever imagined. Choose carefully to avoid two problems: misinformation and too much information. Below are names of several organizations that can help you gather facts. They have websites and printed materials, and can direct families to local resources. The Internet can be a terrific resource, but it can also be overwhelming. Choose a site or two that you like, and then visit regularly. Most important, review all information with a physician to ensure that it is accurate and complete:

- American Parkinson's Disease Association (APDA):
  www.apdaparkinson.org
- American Association of Retired Persons (AARP):
  www.aarp.org
- Movement Disorder Society (MDS):
  www.movementdisorders.org
- National Parkinson Foundation (NPF): www.parkinson.org
- Healthfinder: www.healthfinder.gov (This is a site of the
  U.S. Department of Health and Human Services. It is a

free gateway to reliable consumer health and human services information and includes a list of support and self-
help groups.)

On a practical level, assistance is available in most large met-
ropolitan areas for house cleaning, cooking, and running errands. These services are not covered by insurance but can
be well worth the expense. To find services in your community, contact your local Visiting Nurses Association (VNA). The
VNA is a not-for-profit agency that provides home health care
for people of all ages and with any medical condition. To find
the VNA nearest you, check the local yellow pages or log onto
the website for the Visiting Nurses Association of America, at
www.vnaa.org.

While providing support for the person who has Parkinson's
disease is important, it is equally important that family members recognize their own needs and develop effective coping
strategies. The stress can be considerable when someone you
love is facing a chronic illness. Seek help from other family
members, friends, clergy, medical professionals, psychologists,
and support groups. Maintain social contacts—they'll help you
keep perspective and maintain an emotional balance. Remember that *everyone* in the family functions best when they are
healthy. That means eating a well-balanced diet, engaging in regular exercise, and having regular medical check-ups.

This third case study illustrates problem solving for the
spouse of a woman with Parkinson's disease. He found support
from a variety of sources.

*Paula was diagnosed with Parkinson's disease five years ago. Over
the past year, she's grown more and more self-conscious and anxious
about her tremor, especially out in public. She and her husband,
Trevor, had a long-standing habit of going out every Friday night.*

*Even when their now-grown children were young, Friday was date night. Paula always had a babysitter lined up so that she and Trevor could escape for a quiet dinner at a favorite restaurant. Now, Paula refuses to go out to dinner, parties, or other public events, even with family and friends. Trevor feels cut off from his life-long friends and is extremely frustrated by the change in Paula. They have had several serious arguments about his desire to continue with an active social life.*

*Trevor and Paula spoke to Paula's neurologist, who recommended counseling sessions. Paula stopped attending after just two sessions and contends that she's content with her lifestyle. Trevor, however, established a therapeutic relationship with the psychologist and is able to discuss his fears about Paula's declining health. He also began attending a monthly support group for people with Parkinson's disease and their partners that he had read about on the Internet. There he has found a network of friends with whom he can socialize. These friends share similar concerns and, most important to Trevor, do not expect anyone to participate in the discussion who does not want to.*

This case demonstrates how the partner of a person with Parkinson's disease can successfully manage his or her own stress by establishing healthy relationships with people who understand and empathize with the situation.

## More about Coping Skills

There is no doubt that Parkinson's disease is a challenge. It can bring out the best and the worst in families and friends. Our advice is to take a realistic look at your current coping ability and your coping history. Assess where you need help and develop plans for seeking support. By continuing to read this chapter, you may figure out what kind of coping strategy you generally employ.

Most people who have a chronic disease or who are close to someone with a chronic disease experience some psychological distress. Many, research suggests, do not seek support from professional sources. Instead, they depend on themselves and their family and friends for solving problems and for relieving their stress. Challenges include the following:

- obtaining and following through on treatment and advice
- dealing with emotional reactions like anxiety and depression
- managing the effect of the disease on social networks
- coping with work-related losses
- managing threats to self-esteem

Everyone has a personal style of coping with health problems, but there are a few categories that fit most people.

*Direct problem-solvers* seek out answers and support ("I contacted the National Parkinson Foundation to find out more about the disorder."). *Distancers* try to detach themselves from the problem ("I decided not to think about it."). *Positive thinkers* cope by trying to see the problem as a growth experience ("It has drawn us closer together and made us stronger."). *Avoiders* engage in wishful thinking ("It will hopefully get better."). *Escapers* may become involved in self-destructive behaviors like alcohol or drug abuse or eating disorders.

Which strategy works best? Not avoidance or escape into self-destructive behavior, of course. There is some evidence that coping by avoiding the problem (as with distancers, avoiders, and escapers) creates an increased risk for psychological stress. Better outcomes have been associated with positive and active thinking and behaving. If you have difficulty coping with the challenges presented by Parkinson's disease, seek help from a supportive friend, clergy, or professional counselor. You do not need to struggle alone. The goal, ultimately, is to feel better emotionally in order to cope with a difficult and unpredictable situation.

Support from family and friends can reduce the stress associated with having a chronic disease. Patients with a strong support network often have fewer health and emotional problems. They are more likely to use medical services, take medications, follow medical advice, and cope with the stress associated with their condition. Research has found that different kinds of support—emotional or practical—work best when they are provided by the appropriate resource. The results indicate that emotional support is best received when it comes from a close friend or family member. Information and advice is valued most when the source is considered an expert.

Support groups of people who have similar health problems can be great resources. Studies comparing the well-being of people in support groups with that of people who were on waiting lists for such groups have proven it. Patients in support groups discover ways to cope and often find relief from the stigma attached to their medical problem. In support groups for family members and friends, participants get answers to questions about the disease and learn effective strategies for handling their own emotions and for providing emotional support to others.

# 7

# Preserving Intimacy

The effect of Parkinson's disease on a couple's sexual relationship has historically received very little attention from medical professionals. Maybe this is because Parkinson's disease is mostly a condition of older people who are not in the habit of talking about sex, or maybe it is because doctors don't ask patients about the quality and frequency of their sexual relations. The reason is less important than the fact: sexual activity is infrequent when one member of a couple has Parkinson's disease. We know less about the effect of Parkinson's disease on sexual activity in women than in men.

Low sexual desire or an inability to experience sexual arousal is associated with many chronic diseases, not just Parkinson's disease. Decreased frequency of sexual activity and high rates of sexual dysfunction have been identified in patients with a range of medical conditions including cardiovascular disease, cancer, neurological disease, diabetes, end-stage renal disease, and chronic pain. In Parkinson's disease, according to the National Parkinson Foundation, almost 81 percent of men and 43 percent of women report experiencing diminished sexual activity. The problems with intimate relations in Parkinson's disease can be caused by a variety of organic and psychological factors.

If the public response to sildenafil (Viagra) and other medications for improving sexual function is any indication, then most people consider sex an important aspect of a healthy life. Of course, this is not true for everyone, including some people who are extremely debilitated. But research reveals that even terminally ill cancer patients rate intimacy and tenderness, although not necessarily sexual intercourse, as very important.

Some people with Parkinson's disease worry that sexual intercourse is bad for them. Sex will not, in any way, have a harmful effect on the Parkinson's disease itself. Some people note that their tremor is more pronounced after sex. Sex, like any other strenuous physical activity, can cause a worsening of Parkinsonian symptoms that may last for a few minutes to an hour, depending on the person's level of fatigue. Rest assured that there is NO evidence that this temporary worsening of symptoms has any effect on the course of the disease. Some men with Parkinson's disease have trouble achieving and maintaining an erection. Some women experience vaginal dryness. Some people notice a decrease in the intensity of their orgasms. Discuss your particular circumstances with your physician to determine the possible causes and potential treatments. Remember that there are many treatments available to allow people to continue to enjoy sex regardless of age or the existence of chronic disease.

## Possible Causes of Sexual Dysfunction in Parkinson's Disease

The effect of PD on sexual functioning is a complex topic. The following are some of the possible causes of sexual dysfunction in people with Parkinson's disease:

- physical factors
- psychological factors
- medications
- embarrassment and negative body image
- abnormalities of the autonomic nervous system

- low dopamine levels in the brain
- age and menopause
- loss of dexterity
- dosing schedule for anti-Parkinsonian medications
- miscellaneous factors

Psychological factors that can interfere with a healthy sex life include depression, anxiety, and low self-esteem, to name a few. Depression, for example, is common in Parkinson's disease (and should be addressed with a physician or other trained professional), and certain medications that can help overcome depression have side effects related to reduced interest in sex, low sexual arousal, or the inability to attain an orgasm. This is especially true of some of the selective serotonin reuptake inhibitors (SSRIs, such as Celexa, Prozac, Luvox, Paxil, and Zoloft). If depression is a factor in your circumstances, a skilled professional can work with you and your partner to find the best antidepressant medication with the fewest sexual side effects. Antidepressants work differently in different people, and it can take a little time to find the right medication or combination of medications for your circumstances. People often do see results. For more detailed information about depression and medications, see Chapter 8, "Depression."

Embarrassment can also negatively affect sexual activity. Some people are self-conscious of their Parkinson's symptoms and the problems with grooming and appearance that can arise as a result of the disease.

*Marissa is sixty-four years old and was diagnosed with Parkinson's disease four years ago. She feels lucky that she is still alive, able to continue working and taking long walks on the weekends. However, she is upset that her face has become like a mask, devoid of expression. Marissa no longer likes to pose for pictures, because no matter how happy she is when the picture is taken, she always has a "blank stare" in the photograph. Her husband, Robert, is also upset by her lack of facial expression. Even during their most intimate moments, Marissa appears not to be engaged or enjoying their time together. Marissa didn't realize that Robert was affected by this aspect of her condition until one evening, in the middle of a serious argument that began over something minor, he blurted it out. For several months afterward Marissa was self-conscious and unable to engage in sexual relations. She and Robert then sought the help of a therapist, and began to focus on ways to adapt and continue to enjoy a satisfying physical relationship.*

Convention suggests that women are more affected by appearance than men and that men are more affected by changes in their ability to perform sexually. Negative body image and fear of rejection can undoubtedly have an impact on sexuality. If embarrassment is an issue for you, try to remember that problems with grooming can be managed and that being tender, loving, and nonjudgmental—of yourself and your partner—can make adjusting to the disease more manageable.

Men with Parkinson's disease may also experience erectile dysfunction, commonly known as impotence. Erectile dysfunction refers to a difficulty in obtaining or maintaining an erection satisfactory for sexual intercourse. It affects approximately 30 million men in the United States and is estimated to be 1.6 times more common in men with Parkinson's disease than in other men of the same age. The reason for erectile dysfunction in Parkinson's disease is uncertain but there are a few possible explanations. Impotence might be related to abnormalities in the function of the autonomic nervous system, which is seen in people with Parkinson's disease. It might be related to the low dopamine levels in the brain; experimental evidence suggests that dopamine may play a role in normal sexual functioning, so it stands to reason that the abnormally low dopamine levels seen in people with Parkinson's disease could contribute to sexual problems. Parkinson's disease is most common in older people, and we know that aging can also have an effect on sexual performance. Other factors in sexual dysfunction independent of Parkinson's disease and age are cigarette smoking, alcohol use, diabetes, and high cholesterol.

Women with Parkinson's disease can also experience problems with interest in sexual activity, sexual arousal, and reduced orgasm. A reduction in sexual arousal can interfere with normal vaginal expansion and lubrication, making intercourse uncomfortable. It is important to realize that these symptoms can have other causes, like menopause or depression. Medical treatment for women is available. It includes but is not limited to treatment with the hormones estrogen, progestin, or testosterone. Because of the complexity of sexual function and dysfunction, it is best to seek a medical evaluation to determine the best treatment strategy for you. Although sex can be an embarrassing and difficult topic to talk about, remember that conversations with your physician are private. Many doctors are hesitant to bring up the subject of sex because they don't want to embarrass their patients. But if you can raise the issue, you'll see that he or she is trained to deal with it in a straightforward fashion. In fact, your physician is the best person to help determine what the problems are and then devise solutions to deal with them.

Another complication for sexual activity among Parkinson's patients and their partners is the fact that the disease can affect mobility and dexterity, making it difficult to move around or roll over in bed. This impaired range of motion can make sexual activity difficult. Dosing schedules for anti-Parkinsonian medications can also contribute to sexual problems. Typical drug regimens are designed to produce optimal motor function in the morning. The result is that people experience poorer motor function at night, when they are most likely to feel like being intimate. A simple solution for some people would be to coordinate taking medications with sexual activity.

Difficulty reaching orgasm is not as common in people with chronic disease as are problems with sexual desire or arousal. When problems do exist, they are usually related to a decrease in the intensity of orgasm. Medications, particularly the SSRI antidepressants, can be the cause. High doses of alcohol can also interfere with orgasm.

## If Intimacy Is a Problem

Problems with intimacy, arousal, and sexual activity in someone with a chronic disease can be managed. As with everything else related to the condition, finding a solution requires taking steps that can sometimes seem challenging.

As we've mentioned in this section, the sexual problems could be due to the disease itself, to depression, to medications, or to any number of other factors. Here are several tips for addressing sexual difficulties:

- Involve your partner in any discussions and in any treatment plans. After all, changes in sexual function and activity involve both members of a couple.
- Talk to your doctor, who may recommend that you and your partner make an appointment with a medical specialist to assess the situation. The specialist may be a gynecologist, an endocrinologist who specializes in sexual function, or a urologist.
- Consider getting help from a mental health professional. Patients with sexual difficulties are often referred to a sex therapist for assessment and counseling. Sex therapists have special training in reducing the discomfort that many

people feel about discussing sexual issues; they can also offer specific suggestions to help a couple improve their sexual experience.

It should be obvious to anyone who is reading this book or living with someone with Parkinson's disease that managing the situation requires a lot of knowledge, understanding, patience, and compassion. It also takes trust that both members of a couple will do the best they can under the circumstances. Whether you are dealing with issues surrounding sexual intimacy or anything else, remember that many people benefit from talking with their health care providers and by using community resources to acquire information to help them deal with new emotional and physical challenges.

# 8

# Depression

*Miguel was diagnosed with Parkinson's disease three years ago. At that time, he had a rest tremor involving his left arm, and he complained of constantly feeling tired. He began taking carbidopa/ levodopa (Sinemet) as prescribed by his neurologist and had been doing well. Miguel works as an attorney in a private law firm. He shares a home with Alan, his partner of fourteen years.*

*Alan recently noticed that Miguel was taking longer to perform certain tasks, particularly dressing for work in the morning. He was slower in buttoning his shirt, for example, and knotting his tie. At Alan's insistence, Miguel made an appointment to see their primary care physician, Dr. Blair. They scheduled a time when they could visit the doctor together.*

*During the appointment, Alan revealed that he was spending sleepless nights worrying that he would soon have to help Miguel with very basic tasks. A successful businessman who typically spends one week of every month out of town, Alan was worried that he would have to change jobs in order to be home when Miguel needed him. Alan enjoys his job and was feeling angry toward Miguel. He acknowledged that the anger would quickly turn to guilt and that he would then feel terrible. He was dealing with his feelings by over-eating.*

*It was clear that Alan was not coping well with Miguel's illness. Dr. Blair recommended that Miguel make an appointment with his neurologist, to determine if he would benefit from an adjustment in his Parkinson medications. Dr. Blair also diagnosed Alan with depression. Alan agreed to see both a therapist and a psychiatrist, to establish a treatment plan of therapy, medication, or both, to alleviate his depression.*

Depression is very common among patients with Parkinson's disease. About half of PD patients with depression have a form called dysthymia. This is a common and mild form of depression that, if left untreated, tends to become chronic and long-lasting. A person with dysthymia goes through the day functioning at a less than optimal level. You may recognize the symptoms in your family member with Parkinson's disease or even in yourself. Dysthymia can occur in people of all ages, even young children.

There are many symptoms of dysthymia. Here are some of the thoughts, feelings, and behaviors that people with dysthymia may experience:

- decreased self-esteem
- feelings of guilt
- exaggerated self-critical thoughts
- difficulty concentrating or making decisions
- feelings of hopelessness
- sad mood
- tearful episodes
- a change in eating or sleeping habits
- reckless behavior
- low energy

Dysthymia, while unpleasant, is qualitatively different from major depression.

Major depression is also common in people with Parkinson's disease. The symptoms of major depression are similar to those of dysthymia but more severe. They seriously interfere with a person's ability to work, study, sleep, eat, and enjoy life. An episode of major depression usually lasts for a short period of time, just weeks or a few months. It can occur just once, but people who have had one episode are likely to experience another.

Researchers and clinicians working in the mental health field find unique characteristics of depression in patients with Parkinson's disease. Participants at a 2001 meeting at the National Institutes of Health described how depression in people with Parkinson's disease can be different from depression in the rest of the population. The differences are especially marked, they noted, with respect to three features of depression: anxiety, sadness, and suicide. Parkinson patients with depression experience higher rates of anxiety than the general population, are more often sad without feeling guilt or self-blame, and have lower rates of suicide despite higher rates of suicidal thought.[1]

Despite all that we know about depression, it frequently goes undiagnosed in Parkinson's disease. Patients, families, and even their health care providers might be assuming that the symptoms are part of the Parkinson's syndrome and not separately treatable. In the majority of cases, nothing could be further from the truth.

Depression may be common, but more important, it is also treatable. Because of the recent availability of a wide range of effective antidepressant medications, no one needs to suffer through its uncomfortable symptoms. Many people with depression blame their personality or inner character for their mental health, especially when they are in a low period. It is important to understand that depression has biochemical origins; the reason the newer medications are effective is that they target the problem in the cells of the brain. Taking a medication for depression is no different from taking a medication for high blood pressure or asthma. They all work on the underlying organic cause of the disorder.

## Getting Help

Getting help for depression for someone with Parkinson's disease is important and should be part of every treatment plan. Most people find that treatment not only relieves their symptoms of depression but also helps them cope more effectively with daily life and the changes that they experience physically and mentally as a result of Parkinson's disease. Treatment often includes prescription antidepressant medications and psychological counseling.

Mental health professionals are usually the best source of treatment for depression. A family doctor or neurologist should be able to recommend a psychiatrist, psychologist, or social worker who understands chronic disease. A psychiatrist is an M.D., a medical doctor who received his or her training in a medical school and hospital. A psychologist holds a master's degree or a Ph.D. from a university. In some states you must have a Ph.D. degree to call yourself a psychologist. A social worker usually holds a bachelor's or master's degree from a school of social work and, like a psychologist, could have trained in any number of professional settings.

In nearly every state in the United States, only medical doctors are allowed to prescribe antidepressant medications. Therefore, when psychologists or social workers determine that medication could be helpful, they send the patient to a medical doctor, often a psychiatrist, for evaluation for the most suitable antidepressant.

Fee structures and services differ among professions. Your doctor or insurance carrier should be able to provide a list of professionals from whom you can choose. Most health plans have specific guidelines for mental health coverage, so it's a good idea to check with your insurance company if you're concerned about cost. Ideally, you should select the therapist who best suits your needs by interviewing several different professionals on the telephone or by making appointments for office visits. Most therapists charge a fee for an initial visit, but it is worth it. The interview is an important tool to help ensure that the therapist's philosophy and personal style are a good match for you. If your first choice turns out not to suit your needs, try again until you find someone you like and trust.

Physicians and mental health therapists generally like patients (sometimes referred to as clients by therapists) to ask questions and be involved in decision-making. Here are a few questions that therapists expect prospective patients to ask:

- Are you familiar with Parkinson's disease? If not, have you worked with patients and families dealing with a different chronic disease?
- How do you view your role and the client's role in counseling?
- How active a participant are you? Do you mostly listen or advise?
- Do you give homework assignments?
- What are your credentials?
- What is your educational background and training?
- Please explain your policies about fees and insurance.
- How do you handle missed appointments?
- Would you be talking with my physician to coordinate care?
- How long do you typically work with clients? Weeks? Years?
- Is there anything else you can tell me that would help me understand your therapeutic style?

## Types of Treatment

There are two approaches to treating depression: psychotherapy and antidepressant medications. Some patients do best using both at the same time. Others use one or the other.

## Psychotherapy

Psychotherapies are talk therapies in which patients discuss troubling events in their lives. A patient works with a therapist to understand or change the way he or she reacts to events. Three common styles of psychotherapy are cognitive/behavioral therapy, interpersonal therapy, and psychodynamic therapy. These are general categories, however, and it's important to keep in mind that no two therapists will share the exact same approach. In fact, many therapists mingle elements of all three styles of psychotherapy depending on the needs of the patient. Most talk therapies are weekly and short term, for about ten to twenty weeks. Each therapy session is usually forty-five to fifty minutes long.

*Cognitive/behavior therapy* helps people see how their feelings and behavior can be influenced by the way they think. Say, for example, that you promised to speak to a group of gardeners at your civic organization about the most effective way to prevent bug infestation in tomato plants. It turns out that you have bug problems of your own, but in your stomach—in other words, butterflies. Most people would take this to mean that they are nervous and afraid. Why not excited and eager instead? Notice how the more upbeat adjectives give the stomach sensation a positive and much more pleasant twist. Cognitive/behavior therapy helps patients identify the negative patterns of thinking and behaving that may contribute to their depression.

*Interpersonal therapy* explores a patient's relationships with family, friends, colleagues, and even strangers to find patterns that might be triggering the depression or other negative feelings. This approach assumes that there is a connection between mood and relationships, that something is faulty in the mix, and that mood will improve once the pattern is identified and changes are made.

*Psychodynamic therapy* evolved from the original Freudian style of psychoanalytic therapy, but it is usually of shorter duration than what Freud employed and focuses on a specific problem like depression rather than on the whole personality. The therapist tries to help the patient identify the underlying causes of his or her problem. This psychodynamic approach explores a person's past to learn what events led up to the current emotional state. It assumes that emotions drive actions and that understanding the underlying emotion will allow a person to make changes and eliminate the cause of the depression or other problem.

Psychotherapy works well for many people with Parkinson's disease. It is most effective when the psychotherapist and the patient have a good working relationship and the patient understands that there is effort involved in feeling better. Here are some of the ways psychotherapy is effective for overcoming depression:

- It pinpoints life problems that contribute to depression.
- It explores negative or distorted patterns of thinking and behaving that contribute to feelings of despair and helplessness.
- It helps a person understand which aspects of the problems can be solved or improved.
- It identifies realistic goals for improving emotional well-being.
- It helps people regain a sense of control and pleasure in life.

## Antidepressant Medications

Medications can be very effective in managing depression, particularly when the depression is moderate, severe, or chronic.

Combining talk therapy and antidepressant drugs is a common approach that has been shown to be very effective. Because antidepressant medications take a few weeks to reach maximum effectiveness, they are generally not prescribed for depression that lasts just a few days. (In fact, short-lived unhappiness is by definition not depression. The term *depression* is reserved for symptoms that last for a longer period of time.) People who are diagnosed with dysthymia, the persistent sensation of feeling low and out of sorts, can be excellent candidates for antidepressant medications. So can people whose symptoms continue for several weeks or who are not responding to talk therapy.

The most commonly prescribed antidepressants for people with Parkinson's disease are the selective serotonin reuptake inhibitors (SSRIs). This category includes drugs like fluoxetine (Prozac), sertraline (Zoloft), citalopram (Celexa), paroxetine (Paxil), and fluvoxamine (Luvox). Millions of people worldwide use the SSRIs for depression, and the effect has been quite remarkable. Most report that they feel better and become more productive. In fact, studies indicate that 35–45 percent of people who take an SSRI experience complete resolution of their symptoms. (See Table 3.)

The SSRIs are not perfect, and side effects can limit their use. Not everyone experiences side effects, but those who do might feel like they are simply trading one unpleasant condition for another. Since fluoxetine (Prozac) was introduced in the 1980s, it has become apparent that it and the other SSRI drugs come with their own set of problems, both acute and chronic. Acute side effects—including dry mouth, jumpiness, headache, and stomach distress—tend to be mild and are well tolerated by most people. Longer-lasting (but reversible after the medication is discontinued) adverse effects include weight gain, loss of interest in sex and the inability to achieve orgasm, insomnia, and memory lapses. Not all SSRIs have the same effect in all users, so a doc-

*Table 3*  Antidepressant medications commonly used in Parkinson's
disease patients

| Drug class | Generic name | Brand name |
| --- | --- | --- |
| Selective serotonin reuptake inhibitor (SSRI) | Fluoxetine | Prozac |
| SSRI | Paroxetine | Paxil |
| SSRI | Sertraline | Zoloft |
| SSRI | Fluvoxamine | Luvox |
| SSRI | Citalopram | Celexa |
| Tricyclic antidepressant (TCA) | Amitriptyline | Elavil |
| TCA | Nortriptyline | Pamelor |
| TCA | Imipramine | Tofranil |
| Atypical antidepressant | Venlafaxine | Effexor |
| Atypical antidepressant | Bupropion | Wellbutrin |
| Atypical antidepressant | Mirtazapine | Remeron |

tor usually works closely with a patient to find the one drug that
is most effective with the least number of side effects. There is
no doubt that the drugs work, but it might take some time to
find the one that is right for you or your loved one.

Patients with Parkinson's disease sometimes have problems
tolerating the SSRIs because, unlike the older types of antidepressants, which were sedating, these can be activating. That
can be good news for people who are depressed and withdrawn
but quite the opposite for someone who is agitated. SSRIs can
also be problematic for patients who take selegiline (Deprenyl)
to treat their symptoms of Parkinson's disease. The manufacturers of SSRIs recommend against the combination of an SSRI
and selegiline because of the potential for an adverse biochemical effect. This effect is referred to as the "serotonin syndrome"
and may include irritability, hyperthermia, increased muscle
tone, and altered consciousness. The potential for interactions
among various drugs makes it critical for patients to review all
their medications, whether prescription or over the counter,
with their physician or physicians.

Despite these caveats, doctors do prescribe SSRIs to their patients with Parkinson's disease, and most are satisfied with the outcome. The older antidepressants such as amitriptyline (Elavil) or nortriptyline (Pamelor), which are in a category known as the tricyclic antidepressants, are sometimes prescribed instead of the SSRIs.

In addition, there are several relatively new antidepressant medications that are not classified as either SSRIs or tricyclics. Buproprion (Wellbutrin), for example, is an effective antidepressant. Another alternative for the treatment of depression is mirtazapine (Remeron).

The decision of whether to treat depression and the choice of which antidepressant to use should be made in close consultation with your neurologist and psychiatrist or therapist.

## Other Psychiatric Aspects of Parkinson's Disease

The primary pathology in Parkinson's disease is the degeneration of dopamine-producing cells in the substantia nigra. But other portions of the brain are affected, too, including systems that control emotion and thinking.

*Anna has been treated for Parkinson's disease for four years. She enjoys spending time with her grandchildren and until recently worked part-time in a florist shop. Until two years ago, Anna had an active social life. She would meet friends for lunch once a week, and she and her husband would go out with other couples—many of whom had been their friends since high school—almost every weekend.*

*Anna has slowly stopped all social activities. She quit her job because she felt that standing in the store was "just too much." Whenever she was with customers, she was acutely aware of her tremor and she felt that everyone was staring at her. Anna's last luncheon date with friends was six months ago, when she met several women at one of her favorite restaurants. Once they were seated, Anna felt that the women had noticed her tremor and were staring at her. Anna felt her heart begin to race, she became short of breath, and her face felt hot. She left the restaurant, drove home, and has not eaten out since that day.*

What Anna experienced were symptoms of anxiety, and you may have noticed something similar in your family member who has Parkinson's disease. Anxiety is almost as common as depression in people with Parkinson's disease. In one study, researchers found that 28 percent of patients with PD had an anxiety disorder, and another 40 percent had some symptoms of anxiety.[2] An anxiety disorder, as described by the American Psychiatric Association, refers to a group of illnesses—generalized anxiety disorder, phobias, panic disorders, post-traumatic stress disorder, and obsessive-compulsive disorders—and includes symptoms such as excessive worry, dizziness, tension, diarrhea, and racing heart.

Late in the course of Parkinson's disease some people also lose their ability to anticipate, plan, initiate activities, or inhibit their actions. These acts are referred to as executive functions and are essential for reasoning and decision-making. Abnormalities in executive functioning can lead to difficulties with communication, social interaction, and independence.

*Liz and Tony had been married for forty years. Tony was diagnosed with Parkinson's disease ten years ago. In the past year, he has stopped his daily habit of getting up early to garden or walk. More and more often he simply sits in his chair and watches television. He stopped telephoning friends and no longer seems able to make plans to meet them for lunch or cards.*

Parkinson's disease may also lead to impairment in visuospatial skills, that is, in the ability to process and understand visual information. Driving a car, for example, can become difficult and even dangerous because of a person's slowed response time and difficulty interpreting what is happening on the road ahead. Rather than waiting for an accident to occur that might result in injury to you, your passengers, or others, consider undergoing a comprehensive driving evaluation. Some rehabilitation centers offer such evaluations. Keep in mind, though, that the cost of the evaluation is typically not covered by insurance. Giving up the right to drive a car is a difficult step and usually means increased dependence on family and friends, but it is a good choice when the circumstances require it.

*Tip:* If you begin to suspect that you or your loved one is experiencing a decline in executive function and visuospatial skills, point this out to the doctor, who can test to determine the extent of the decline and make helpful recommendations.

Even the drugs that are prescribed to relieve the motor symptoms of Parkinson's disease can cause psychological problems. Their job, after all, is to alter brain chemistry. As drug doses increase to ease worsening motor symptoms, the effect on behavior and mood can become especially evident. Some people may experience hallucinations, delusions, agitation, mania, or confusion.

Visual hallucinations are a common side effect of medications used to treat Parkinson's disease. Some people describe auditory and tactile hallucinations, too, meaning that they hear nonexistent sounds and feel sensations that can't be attributed to real stimuli.

We don't know for sure how many people with PD experience hallucinations, but it may be about 30 percent. Hallucinations are most common in older people who are taking high doses of anti-Parkinsonian drugs and who have some cognitive impairment.

Visual hallucinations usually occur at night and are typically non-threatening. In fact, family members are sometimes surprised when the topic of hallucinations comes up and their loved one mentions seeing people or animals that they know do not exist. Patients often understand that their hallucinations are a side effect of the medication, and many are willing to live with them. When side effects are troubling, a doctor will usually try to eliminate or reduce them by altering the dose of medication. There are also numerous medications that, in relatively small doses, can control the hallucinations quite well.

Delusions in Parkinson's disease usually manifest as a fear of being injured, poisoned, followed or watched, deceived, or unfairly influenced. The number of people with Parkinson's disease who experience delusions from medication is estimated to be between 3 and 17 percent.

Agitation is another psychiatric condition that can occur in PD patients. Agitation refers to uncharacteristic stubbornness, worrying, and nervousness. Signs of agitation might include irritability, repetitive questioning, refusal to cooperate, pacing, and yelling. Agitation can sometimes be managed by simplifying tasks or finding an interesting distraction for the patient.

Medications for Parkinson's disease have also been associated with mania. The characteristics of mania include euphoria, a feeling of high self-esteem, increased psychomotor activity, exuberance, a diminished need for sleep, and hypersexuality (the exhibition of unusual or excessive concern with or indulgence in sexual activity).

Hallucinations, delusions, agitation, or mania do not occur in everyone with Parkinson's disease. For those who do suffer from these side effects, lowering the dose of the drug usually makes the symptoms subside. The doctor and patient must weigh the benefit of changing drug dosages because there is always a trade-off. Lowering the dose will undoubtedly cause a return of the motor symptoms of Parkinson's disease. Alternatively, add-

*Table 4*   Atypical antipsychotic medications commonly
used in Parkinson's disease patients

| Generic name | Brand name |
| --- | --- |
| Clozapine | Clozaril |
| Quetiapine | Seraquel |
| Risperidone | Risperdal |

ing a low dose of one of the newer antipsychotic drugs, referred to as "atypical" antipsychotics, can be quite effective in controlling the behavioral problems without worsening the motor symptoms associated with Parkinson's disease. Unlike the older antipsychotics, the newer, atypical antipsychotics have a lesser risk of worsening the signs and symptoms of Parkinson's disease. Thus, a low dose of an atypical antipsychotic medicine can control behavior without making someone with Parkinson's disease slower or more rigid. Confusion and agitation in someone with Parkinson's disease can take a tremendous toll on the entire family, and it is important to remember that this behavior can be controlled with medication. (See Table 4.)

## Depression Preceding the Onset of PD Symptoms

Like the whistle blast that signals a train coming around the bend, so can depression be a prelude to Parkinson's disease. This is not to say that depression is a risk factor for Parkinson's disease. Hardly. The number of people in the United States who suffer from depression, according to the National Institute of Mental Health, is about 18.8 million in any given year, compared with the number of people with Parkinson's disease, which is many times less at 1.2 million in North America. Nonetheless, in looking back at their mental health before the motor signs of their Parkinson's disease developed, many patients report symptoms of depression. Researchers think that the depression is probably caused by lower levels of the chemical serotonin in the brain. Studies have shown that people with Parkinson's disease have a lowered level of serotonin.

Serotonin is a neurotransmitter that is released from certain nerve cells to stimulate other nerve cells. When it is absent or not working effectively, a person experiences depression. Normally, serotonin is released from a cell, stimulates other nerve cells, and then returns to a serotonin-producing cell to be repackaged and released again to do its work. Hence, the logic behind the antidepressant medications called selective serotonin reuptake inhibitors (SSRIs). When quantities of serotonin are low, the SSRIs prevent the return (reuptake) of the chemical so that its effect lasts longer at the second cell and a normal string of events in the brain can be maintained.

Serotonin has another function: It also modulates the release of dopamine, which, as we know, at low levels is responsible for the rigidity and tremor of Parkinson's disease. Researchers believe that a decrease in serotonin might be caused by the low levels of dopamine in people with Parkinson's disease. This suggests a feedback mechanism between the brain cells that produce serotonin and those that produce dopamine.

In biological systems we often see feedback loops, in which one biological event (say, a cell's production of a particular chemical) is influenced by an earlier event (say, the presence or absence of another chemical). In the system suggested here, low levels of dopamine "tell" the serotonin-producing cells to produce less serotonin. With less serotonin, a person's chance of developing depression increases. Does this mean that if you are depressed, you are at risk for Parkinson's disease? There is no evidence that depression causes Parkinson's disease; we just know that depression in people who end up with Parkinson's disease may be an early symptom of the disorder.

In 2002, convincing research supporting this link between depression and Parkinson's disease was published in a scientific journal called *Neurology* and presented at a meeting of the American Academy of Neurology. The researchers began with a health directory containing medical information about all the patients seen by general practitioners in fifty-three different medical practices in the Netherlands. They identified the patients who had symptoms of depression. The health directory contained records of nearly 69,000 people. Of this group, 1,358 fit the strict criteria for depression established for this study. They could not be psychotic and must have experienced at least three of the following six feelings:

1. sadness or melancholy more than can be explained by psychosocial stress
2. suicidal thoughts or attempts
3. indecisiveness, decreased interest in usual activities, or diminished ability to think
4. feelings of worthlessness, self-reproach, or inappropriate or excessive guilt
5. early morning awakening, excessive sleeping, or early morning fatigue
6. anxiety, extreme irritability, or agitation

How many in the depressed group developed Parkinson's disease? The answer was 19. How many from the nondepressed group developed Parkinson's disease? The researchers discovered 259. Converting to percentages, 1.4 percent of people in the depressed group developed Parkinson's disease compared with 0.4 percent in the nondepressed group. This might not sound like much of a difference, but in epidemiological terms the results reveal a significant connection between Parkinson's disease and depression.[3]

## More on Parkinson's Disease and Mental Health

Patients, families, and doctors often notice a correlation between "off" periods and depression. An "off" period, again, is when there is not enough dopamine in a person's blood and brain to allow that person to function at his or her normal capacity. Movements become slow and stiff. Tremor and episodes of freezing may be increased.

Other symptoms of Parkinson's disease can be confused with depression. These include anergy (lack of energy), anhedonia (inability to experience pleasure), apathy (lack of emotion or caring), and passivity (disinterest in participating in an activity). Hypomimia (expressionless face), hypophonia (soft voice), and slow walk in Parkinson's disease can also be mistaken for depression. If you have any concerns about your diagnosis, speak with your doctor or get a second opinion.

# 9

# Dementia

Some families worry that Parkinson's disease will cause dementia. In many cases the fear of dementia is so great that people
are afraid to ask about it. Remember, knowledge is your best
weapon against Parkinson's disease or any other chronic illness.
Gathering information by reading and asking questions of the
physicians on your or your loved one's treatment team is the
best way to learn about and cope with the varied symptoms of
Parkinson's disease.

Most people think of PD as a condition that affects just physical movement. But as we have shown in this book, Parkinson's
disease can have an impact on many different areas of life. In
this chapter, we address dementia and cognitive function, perhaps the area of greatest concern to those who have just been diagnosed with PD and their loved ones. We discuss several reports from the medical literature concerning cognitive function
in patients with Parkinson's disease. The word *cognition* refers to
the mental processes that a person employs in the gathering and
use of information.

Families who ask about dementia usually want to know if they
will see the same kind of decline in cognitive function that we
usually associate with Alzheimer's disease. Mostly, they want to
know if Parkinson's disease will affect thinking, speech, and behavior. The simplest answer to this question is that research
shows that some patients with Parkinson's disease perform less

well on cognitive tests than their age-matched controls (generally meaning healthy people of the same age, race, gender, and educational level). The pattern of cognitive changes in Parkinson's disease, however, is not the same as in Alzheimer's disease, which may reflect a difference in the brain region that is affected by the two diseases.

It's important to keep in mind that muscles of the head and neck are not spared in Parkinson's disease. Thus the face of a person with Parkinson's disease will not reflect emotions as clearly and as quickly as it once did. Moreover, the muscles that are responsible for swallowing do not work as efficiently, and saliva that is ordinarily swallowed can build up in the mouth, which can result in drooling. These symptoms of Parkinson's disease should *not* be confused with dementia.

## Dementia and Cognitive Function Defined

The term *dementia* refers to a clinical syndrome in which there is a decline of mental ability owing to alterations in the structure or activity of the brain. The onset of dementia is usually slow, and it is associated with many different medical disorders. There are also different types of dementia; the portion of the brain that is affected will determine what kinds of behavioral characteristics and changes in cognitive function a person will experience.

Cognitive function refers to the capacity of an individual to perform tasks that require the gathering of information and the integration of that information into a useful whole. When James Parkinson originally described the disease that came to be named after him, he believed that patients experienced no cognitive loss. We now know that this is incorrect. Some patients with Parkinson's disease do experience a decline in cognitive function. Many psychological tests are available to measure the degree of decline in cognitive ability and the type of functions that are compromised.

When evaluating a person's cognitive function, doctors generally consider several areas. These cognitive "domains" include attention, memory, executive functions, visuospatial functions, verbal functions, and thinking and reasoning.

Research indicates that some cognitive domains are more likely than others to be affected by Parkinson's disease. Those most often affected are attention, memory and learning, executive functions, and visuospatial functions. Verbal function and thinking and reasoning seem to be spared, although information processing may be slower than before the onset of the disease. Slowed information processing is referred to as brady-phrenia, with *brady-* meaning slow (as in bradykinesia, or slow movement) and *-phrenia* referring to the head.

*Attention* is the ability to focus and concentrate on a designated stimulus, sensation, idea, or thought. It can apply to the ability to focus and concentrate on things that are presented visually or verbally. Attention and concentration are important to cognitive functioning because things such as memory and planning require us to pay attention.

*Memory* refers to the store of knowledge that we acquire through experience. In Parkinson's disease, something called *free recall* is impaired while another type of memory referred to as *cued recall* remains largely intact. Free recall is also referred to as active memory. An example of free recall would be the ability to tell someone what you did today or the names of your grandchildren. An example of cued recall, or passive memory, would be the ability to point to your grandchild in a group photograph.

*Executive functions* are mental processes involved in goal-directed behavior. People with Parkinson's disease generally have problems with internally guided behavior but manage just fine when behavior is externally guided. What does this mean in practical terms? For example, a person with PD might have difficulty deciding that he or she is hungry and that pizza sounds appetizing, and then managing the operations involved in having the pizza delivered. On the other hand, that same person might have no trouble following instructions to look up the telephone number of the pizza shop, to call the shop, and then to order the pizza. The latter is an example of externally guided behavior.

Other executive functions, like attaining an "attentional set" (for example, deciding to pull weeds in the garden and actually doing it) and "set shifting" (moving between two closely related tasks, like pulling weeds and picking beans from the same garden without mixing the two in the same pail) may also be affected.

*Visuospatial functions* refer to the ability to process and understand visual information. Assessment of visuospatial and visuoconstructive skills is difficult in patients with motor impairment, but motor-free tasks suggest that those with Parkinson's disease have visuospatial deficits distinct from their motor abnormalities. Examples of visuospatial and visuoconstructive skills in everyday life are drawing a map showing how to get from your house to the grocery store, setting the table for dinner, and tying shoelaces.

Researchers and clinicians typically measure these cognitive functions by using paper and pencil tests or by having a person take the tests on a computer. Testing of cognitive function is usually performed by a specially trained psychologist and takes a couple of hours. The psychologist explains in general terms what the patient will be doing during the testing session and then interviews the patient to learn about past and current life events, health problems, and so on. Then the testing begins with tasks that are varied in type and intensity. The patient is asked to answer some questions verbally while others require putting puzzles together or arranging blocks to match a drawing. Reading and writing tasks may also be part of the testing. Sometimes the psychologist will ask the patient to take a test that involves using a computer. Tasks are usually alternated to keep the testing interesting. For example, a reading task might be followed by puzzles followed by questions from the psychologist. Some tasks are timed while others are open-ended. Certain tasks are very easy and others are very difficult in order to challenge the full range of the patient's abilities.

During the testing the psychologist encourages the patient to do his or her best, but does not reveal scores, correct answers, or any observations. Many people find the testing interesting and entertaining. No one gets all the questions or tasks right all the time. The results are usually shared with the patient and, if the patient or an appointed family member approves, designated members of the medical team and other family members.

## Statistics

In a study of Parkinson's patients in Great Britain who were newly diagnosed with the disease, researchers found that 36 percent showed some form of cognitive impairment.[1] The researchers used well-established, standardized psychological tests to measure a variety of cognitive domains. The total number of patients included in the study was 159, ranging in age at the time of their diagnosis from about 38 to 90. Of the group, 57 showed some form of cognitive impairment. Thirteen of the 57 had evidence of a high degree of cognitive impairment.

This British study agrees with the findings of another study, conducted in the United States, estimating that 20–40 percent of patients with Parkinson's disease experience some degree of cognitive loss.[2]

## What Could Be Causing the Changes?

This is another difficult question. The answer is probably that the different forms of cognitive change are related to a decrease in the normal function of the different sections of the brain related to these functions. Low scores on tests related to memory would be linked to changes in one part of the brain, for example, whereas alterations in thinking and reasoning would be linked to another.

The connection between cognitive loss and brain region was demonstrated in the British study mentioned above. Although 57 of the Parkinson's disease patients in the study showed signs of cognitive impairment, they did not all show identical signs. The different tests that the researchers had the patients take were all designed to pinpoint regions of the brain responsible for different behaviors. Thus, for the 12 patients who scored poorly on a test of pattern recognition, the test indicated that the impairment was linked to the region of the brain called the temporal lobe, where the ability to perform pattern recognition tasks is known to reside. In the 17 patients who performed poorly on tests that measure the ability to plan on the basis of working memory, the test indicated that they had a decrease in functioning in the frontostriatal system of the brain. The frontostriatal system is a network of brain cells that extend between the frontal cortex and the striatum, which is part of the basal ganglia. Some Parkinson's disease patients showed signs of impairment in both regions; the patients in this group were significantly older than the other study participants.

Radiology studies (such as positron emission tomography, or PET scans) that allow researchers to observe the brain activity of Parkinson's disease patients reinforce the findings of the psychological tests. PET scans study the brain's blood flow and its metabolism of glucose. Metabolism is a normal and ongoing process in the body for breaking down nutrients to make the energy that cells need to perform their normal, healthy functions. A decrease in glucose metabolism in certain regions of the brain can indicate a malfunction.

PET scans are used in many research studies, but they are not available as part of a routine clinical evaluation. Individuals who agree to participate in a research study that includes PET scans are injected with a mildly radioactive substance that is attached to a material like glucose. The radioactive glucose then transmits a signal as it flows through the bloodstream to various organs, including the brain. A special camera picks up the signal and converts it into an image that we recognize.

Recent PET imaging studies have shown decreased glucose metabolism in the temporal lobe in some patients with Parkinson's disease.[3] Remember that the ability to recognize patterns, a requirement for learning and memory, is governed by the temporal lobe.

In sum, the most commonly identified cognitive problems in people with Parkinson's disease are decreases in attention, memory, executive functions, and visuospatial functions. Language, the ability to recognize people and things, thinking, and reasoning tend to be less affected or unaffected by Parkinson's disease.

## Treatment of Dementia Associated With PD

If your loved one is struggling with Parkinson's-related dementia, ask his or her doctor for help in managing the symptoms. There are drug treatments that control some of the symptoms of dementia in some patients.

Dementia in Parkinson's disease is sometimes attributed not so much to the reduction of dopamine in the brain as to a de-

*Is Parkinson's Dementia the Same as Alzheimer's Dementia?*
Many families ask if the dementia associated with Parkinson's disease is similar to Alzheimer's disease. The answer is generally no. Brain function in Parkinson's disease differs from that seen in Alzheimer's disease. In PD, attention, memory and learning, executive functions, and visuospatial functions are the areas usually affected. Language, thinking, and reasoning typically remain intact.

crease in a different neurotransmitter called acetylcholine. This explains why dopamine therapy has very little effect on cognitive function in Parkinson's disease. For Parkinson's patients with dementia, it thus often makes sense to try acetylcholine-enhancing drugs, particularly those called cholinesterase inhibitors, which prevent the inactivation of the acetylcholine neurotransmitter after it is released from the neuron, allowing it to act for a longer time in the brain. But managing symptoms of dementia in such patients can be complicated and difficult because of potential interactions with other drugs the patients might be taking and the possibility of increasing some physical symptoms while trying to eliminate those related to dementia. Your or your loved one's doctor should evaluate the medications currently being used because some Parkinson's disease medications can contribute to confusion. The doctor will probably withdraw non-essential medications from the patient's regime slowly and in a particular order, to look for signs of improvement.

If no improvement occurs as the regular medications are adjusted, then the acetylcholine-enhancing drugs may be recommended. The four most common anticholinesterase medications are rivastigmine, donepezil, galantamine, and tacrine. The last one, tacrine, is rarely prescribed any more because it can cause liver damage. These medications have been extensively tested and approved for use in people with Alzheimer's dementia. It is not yet clear if they are helpful for the treatment of the cognitive decline seen in those with Parkinson's disease.

The fact that we devote an entire chapter to the topic of cognitive decline in those with Parkinson's disease may seem frightening. It is important to remember that dementia does not come to everyone with PD. But cognitive issues do occur in some people with Parkinson's disease. Your best defense is to become educated and aware of potential problems. Should your loved one develop cognitive problems, remember that you are not alone. Support is available not only from family members, clergy, and Parkinson's disease organizations, but also from agencies devoted specifically to helping those with dementia.

# 10

## Alternative Therapies

Alternative therapies are popular the world over. Their use is quite common among people with Parkinson's disease. This chapter will help you understand several of the most common alternative therapies and how they may affect PD symptoms such as muscle stiffness, depression, and postural instability.

We recommend that you always talk with a physician about the use of alternative therapies. At the end of this chapter we provide a list of questions to ask your doctor, to ensure that the alternative treatment is being used properly and to the best advantage.

### What Is Alternative Therapy?

The answer to this question depends on who you ask. The authors of an article published in the *New England Journal of Medicine* in 1998 define alternative therapy as follows:

> What most sets alternative medicine apart, in our view, is that it is not scientifically tested and its advocates largely deny the need for such testing. By testing, we mean the marshalling of rigorous evidence of safety and efficacy, as required by the Food and Drug Administration for the approval of drugs, by the best peer-reviewed medical journals for the publication of research reports.[1]

The authors of an article in the journal *Neurology* define alternative therapy more simply, as "a treatment based primarily on belief rather than scientific proof of efficacy."[2] The National Institutes of Health divides the practice into two parts: complementary medicine and alternative medicine. They have named a research and funding center accordingly: The National Center for Complementary and Alternative Medicine (NCCAM). Complementary and alternative medicine (CAM) is, as defined by NCCAM,

> a group of diverse medical and health care systems, practices, and products that are not presently considered to be part of conventional medicine . . . while some scientific evidence exists regarding some CAM therapies, for most there are key questions that are yet to be answered through well-designed scientific studies—questions such as whether they are safe and whether they work for the diseases or medical conditions for which they are used.[3]

Complementary medicine, according to NCCAM, is used in conjunction with conventional Western-style medicine. Alternative medicine, in contrast, is a substitute for traditional medicine. An example of alternative medicine might be a special diet to fight cancer in place of radiation, surgery, or chemotherapy.

NCCAM uses the term "integrative medicine" to describe the practice of combining Western-style medicine with CAM therapies for which there is reasonable scientific proof.

## Alternative Therapy in Parkinson's Disease

People with Parkinson's disease frequently use alternative therapy. A study of 201 patients by doctors at Johns Hopkins Medical School and Boston University School of Medicine found that 40 percent had used some form of alternative therapy in conjunc-

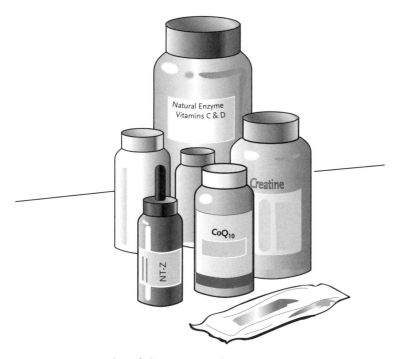

FIGURE 12.    Examples of alternative medicines. Many vitamins and dietary supplements are available over the counter, $CoQ_{10}$ and creatine being just two. It is important to review the use of these agents, just as you would prescription medications, with your doctor. It is a good habit to bring these bottles to your doctor's appointment, so that the two of you can review your use of them together.

tion with traditional treatment. More than 70 percent of this group used more than one form, mostly vitamins and herbs, massage, and acupuncture.

There are many examples of alternative therapies. Several of the most mainstream therapies are described here, including vitamin E, coenzyme $Q_{10}$, massage, St. John's wort, and Chinese exercise modalities. (See Figure 12.)

*Table 5*   Potential interactions of herbs and drugs used as alternative
            therapies by some patients to treat their Parkinson's disease

| Drug combination | Potential adverse reaction |
| --- | --- |
| Pyridoxine (vitamin B6) and carbidopa/levodopa (Sinemet) | Limited absorption of carbidopa/levodopa in the stomach |
| St. John's wort and selegiline (Deprenyl) | Severe hypertension, seizure |

## Vitamins

Recently, a good deal of attention has been given to the use of vitamin supplements for the treatment or prevention of a variety of diseases. There is no solid, overwhelming evidence supporting the benefit of taking any specific vitamin or vitamin combination for the treatment of Parkinson's disease. In fact, taking excess amounts of some vitamins has been found to interfere with the effectiveness of some anti-Parkinsonian medications. For example, vitamin B6 (pyridoxine) at doses of 10 milligrams a day or higher can accelerate the breakdown of levodopa in the body, making it less effective. However, taking one multivitamin a day will not have any deleterious effect on Parkinson's disease and may have some benefit in maintaining overall health. To ensure that vitamin supplements are not harmful, discuss the use of all prescription and nonprescription pills with your physician. (See Table 5.)

### VITAMIN E

Vitamin E belongs to a class of vitamins called antioxidants. The scientific name of vitamin E is tocopherol. Antioxidants fight against free radicals, highly reactive chemical species that arise naturally in the body and brain during normal metabolism. Under certain conditions, free radicals increase in number and can damage cell membranes and their many working parts. Fortunately, the body has developed ways to control free radicals—antioxidants, among them.

In patients with Parkinson's disease and several other neurodegenerative diseases, scientists have detected an increase in cell damage that they blame on an excess of free radicals. They have been looking at the role of vitamin E, which occurs naturally in many foods and is also available as a food supplement, in boosting the brain's ability to fight free radicals as a way to prevent the progression of Parkinson's disease.

Vitamin E initially generated a lot of excitement. In fact, the National Institute of Neurological Disorders and Stroke (NINDS) undertook a major study ("Deprenyl and Tocopherol Antioxidative Therapy for Parkinson's Disease," or DATATOP) to look at the effects of deprenyl (also called selegeline) and vitamin E on early Parkinson's disease. The study involved more than fifty investigators over a five-year period. The results did not provide any evidence that vitamin E helped to slow the early progression of Parkinson's disease.

Despite the findings of the DATATOP study, some scientists still hypothesize that vitamin E or a different antioxidant might be beneficial for people with Parkinson's disease. Vitamin E does not enter the brain easily. Perhaps, some speculate, if the dose were altered or the blood-brain barrier could be breached, the outcome would be different. The blood-brain barrier is a special, highly selective screen that protects the brain from many substances that are in the blood. The brain is nourished by very small blood vessels, called capillaries, that are surrounded by a layer of cells that are all very closely attached. The blood-brain barrier is like a very fine sieve; only very small molecules can cross this layer and actually enter the brain.

Vitamin E can interfere with anticoagulant medicines and,

in high doses, can cause side effects. Vitamin E supplements should be taken only after consultation with your physician.

## COENZYME $Q_{10}$

Coenzyme $Q_{10}$ (also known as $CoQ_{10}$, $Q_{10}$, vitamin $Q_{10}$, ubiquinone, or ubidecarenone) is made naturally by the body. Like vitamin E, coenzyme $Q_{10}$ is an antioxidant, meaning that it protects cells from the damaging effects of free radicals. Coenzyme $Q_{10}$ also helps cells produce the energy they need for normal growth and maintenance. Researchers are taking a serious look at coenzyme $Q_{10}$ because it shows promising signs of being able to slow the decline of patients with Parkinson's disease.

Coenzyme $Q_{10}$ is present in most places in the body, especially the heart, liver, kidneys, and pancreas. Patients with Parkinson's disease, researchers have discovered, have reduced levels of coenzyme $Q_{10}$ in specialized structures inside cells called mitochondria. Recall that mitochondria are necessary for the production of energy in cells. Without energy, cells cannot meet their commitment to the body, whether it is to produce a protein, to repair itself, or to perform some other function.

In a study with a total of eighty subjects, researchers from the University of California at San Diego gave twenty participants a daily dose of 1200 milligrams of coenzyme $Q_{10}$ for a sixteen-month period. They found that these individuals scored significantly better on a Parkinson's disease rating scale at the end of the sixteen-month period than those patients who took either a lower dose of coenzyme $Q_{10}$ or a placebo (a tablet with no biological effects, commonly known as a "sugar pill"). Their rating scale measured mental function and mood, activities of daily living, and motor skills. As the researchers emphasize, this was a small study. An ongoing study of a larger group of patients is exploring whether coenzyme $Q_{10}$ is truly effective in slowing the progression of Parkinson's disease.[4]

Anyone who is considering using coenzyme $Q_{10}$ should talk with his or her physician. Not all food supplements are safe. Coenzyme $Q_{10}$ can interact with certain prescription medicines, which can reduce the effect of the supplement or the medication. For example, coenzyme $Q_{10}$ can alter the body's response to insulin and certain blood-thinning medicines. Nor is it cheap: One year of daily treatment with 1200 milligrams of coenzyme $Q_{10}$ costs at least \$2,400. Most insurance companies do not cover the cost of coenzyme $Q_{10}$ or other CAM medications.

## Marijuana

There has been much discussion in the popular media regarding the medical use of marijuana. A comprehensive, scientific evaluation of the possible therapeutic benefits to Parkinson's patients of cannabis, the active ingredient in marijuana, is in its infancy. In particular, preliminary studies have been done on the use of marijuana in controlling dyskinesias. A recent study to determine the effects of an oral medication that contains cannabis showed that it was safe and well tolerated by Parkinson's patients. However, there is not yet any solid evidence to support the notion that cannabis is helpful in relieving any of the symptoms of Parkinson's disease.

## Massage

The American Massage Therapy Association (AMTA) defines massage therapy as "a profession in which the practitioner applies manual techniques . . . with the intention of positively affecting the health and well-being of the client. Massage is manual soft tissue manipulation."[5]

According to AMTA surveys, massage therapy is growing in-

creasingly popular. From 1997 to 2001, the number of adults re-
porting that they had one or more massages in the previous year
grew from 17 percent to 27 percent. Massage is most popular among people ages 25 to 34, but all age groups are using it
more. In the 55–64 age group, use of massage therapy jumped
from 13 percent to 20 percent in 2000–2001. The study by Johns
Hopkins and Boston University researchers of alternative therapies use among Parkinson patients found that 14 percent had
used massage therapy.

Does massage therapy benefit people with Parkinson's disease? Some patients say that it helps relieve their muscle stiffness and that it provides relaxation physically and mentally. Biologically, massage therapy claims to reduce heart rate, increase
blood and lymph circulation in muscles, relax muscles, reduce
soreness, improve range of motion, and increase endorphins.
These claims have yet to be proven in rigorous, scientific trials.
NCCAM is studying the benefits of massage in cancer, depression, and low back pain.

The most common type of massage therapy is the soothing
Swedish massage. The therapist uses long strokes and knead-
ing and friction techniques to stimulate surface muscles. The
massage is combined with active and passive movement of the
joints. Some types of massage like Rolfing or sports massage
use deep-muscle massage techniques and can even be somewhat painful. The Eastern-based massage therapies Shiatsu and
acupressure use finger pressure to stimulate channels of energy
flow throughout the body.

Massage therapy instruction is rigorous and usually requires
a minimum of five hundred hours of academic and technical
training. The American Massage Therapy Association recom-
mends asking the following questions of a massage therapist before enlisting his or her services:

- Are you currently licensed as a massage therapist in this state/municipality? (Thirty states and the District of Columbia currently require licensing of massage therapists.)
- Are you certified by the National Certification Board for Therapeutic Massage and Bodywork?
- Are you a graduate of a training program accredited by the Commission on Massage Therapy Accreditation, or that is a current AMTA school member?
- Do you have advanced training in any specific massage techniques?

Some but not all insurance companies cover services provided by a massage therapist.

## St. John's Wort

Many people use St. John's wort, an extract derived from a plant (*Hypericum perforatum*), as an alternative therapy for treating their depression. It is one of the best-selling herbal products in the United States. Evidence indicates that it contains chemicals that act like several commonly prescribed antidepressant medications, the serotonin reuptake inhibitors (SSRIs, like Prozac; see Chapter 8).

Does St. John's wort relieve depression? Some say yes. It is widely prescribed in Europe, and a study published in 1996 in the *British Medical Journal* looking at the outcome of twenty-three other studies of St. John's wort found that against mild to moderate depression it works better than a placebo. The choice as to who gets a placebo and who gets the active compound is made randomly. In well-designed clinical trials, neither the study subject nor the physicians evaluating the patients know who is getting what until the trial is completed and the results are analyzed. This type of clinical trial is referred to as "double-blind."

In major depression, however, St. John's wort does not appear to be effective. In a 2002 article in the *Journal of the American Medical Association,* researchers reported different results in patients with major depression. They compared St. John's wort with a placebo and with a prescription SSRI. They found that patients taking a placebo or St. John's wort experienced some improvement in their depression. A bigger difference showed up, though, when these groups were compared with people given SSRIs; the SSRI group improved much more.

People who are thinking of taking St. John's wort should consider these research findings and the risks associated with untreated depression. The U.S. Food and Drug Administration classifies St. John's wort, like vitamins, as a dietary supplement. This means that it can be sold without meeting requirements for safety and effectiveness. Talk with your physician about all dietary supplements and other alternative therapies you are using or thinking of using. Some medications may be adversely affected by St. John's wort and other herbal compounds.


## Chinese Exercise Modalities

Poor balance (postural instability) is one of the hallmark symptoms of Parkinson's disease. Given that PD is a disorder of the motor system of the body, it is not surprising that balance is affected.

Balance disorders can easily lead to falls. Fear of falling and injuries from falls affect independence, so there has been a great deal of research done with elderly people to find effective fall prevention interventions. Exercise to maintain muscle mass has proven to be one effective strategy. Walking is highly recommended; it helps strengthen the muscles that surround the joints, which then act as natural girdles to help keep the joints from giving way.

Physical activity is important because muscles and nerves need constant reminders about their role in keeping us moving and balanced. Most people have had the uncomfortable experience of being unsteady on their feet after a prolonged period of inactivity. Physical activity needn't be as extreme as a vigorous run or weight training; any form of exercise is better than none.

However, it is possible that for people with Parkinson's disease, some types of exercise are even better than other types. Some activities have the benefit of improving not only physical fitness (for example, muscle strength) but also motor control. Studies comparing Chinese exercise modalities to aerobic exercise training may provide an explanation for why this is the case.

Tai chi has become an increasingly popular exercise in the United States and around the world. It is the ancient Chinese martial art whereby slow, graceful movements of the body are coordinated with measured breathing. Tai chi is said to enhance balance, flexibility, cardiovascular fitness, and relaxation. It has also been shown to decrease falls and increase confidence in the elderly. When researchers from Emory University compared falls in two hundred elderly men and women who were given lessons in either tai chi or another form of balance training, they found that the tai chi participants not only decreased their risk of multiple falls by 47.5 percent but also showed greater confidence in their ability to avoid falls.[6]

In 2002, the National Institutes of Health began recruiting people with Parkinson's disease to participate in a study comparing tai chi and walk-run types of exercise. If the people in the group doing standard aerobic exercise perform better on tests of balance than those doing tai chi, then the researchers will assume that the major benefit to Parkinson's disease patients comes from building muscle strength. If people in the tai chi group do as well or better than the aerobic exercise group, this will suggest that there is another beneficial mechanism at work, perhaps a change in the motor-control system of the brain.

Many fitness centers, rehabilitation centers, community centers, and martial arts studios offer lessons in tai chi. The best way to learn tai chi is from an experienced instructor. Helpful books and videos are also available. It is always a good idea to discuss plans to use any form of supplemental treatment or exercise program with your physician before beginning.

## Use Caution

Understandably, people with chronic disease are often eager to find ways to relieve their discomfort. For relief from the symptoms of Parkinson's disease, a fairly long list of vitamins, herbs, diets, and other substances and techniques have evolved. If you are considering alternative therapies, follow the advice of the National Center for Complementary and Alternative Medicine and ask your physician for answers to the following questions:

- What benefits can be expected from this therapy?
- What are the risks associated with this therapy?
- Do the known benefits outweigh the risks?
- What side effects can be expected?
- Will the therapy interfere with conventional treatment?
- Is this therapy part of a clinical trial? If so, who is sponsoring the trial?
- Will the therapy be covered by health insurance?

Alternative therapies may be helpful for some people, but not for everyone. Some therapies may even be dangerous. A major concern among doctors is the fact that most patients do not tell them about the alternative therapies they are using. It is important to maintain open, honest lines of communication with your doctor. Families, friends, and the media can be good sources of information about alternative therapies, but you should always consult your physician to ensure that the information is correct, and that the therapy you're considering is safe for you. By telling your doctor all the medications you're taking, you can avoid potentially serious complications from the interactions between traditional prescription medication and alternative treatments. And most important, establishing an open dialog with your physician will help both of you determine the best course of treatment. The questions recommended by NCCAM will help build trust between you and your doctor.

# 11

# Clinical Trials

*Antonio turned on his television set to hear the latest financial reports and to find out how the stock market had done that day. Suddenly, he was pulled in by a report about a small biotechnology company with a new drug that the reporter was saying might be a treatment for Parkinson's disease. Of course, the television analysts were focusing on how FDA (Food and Drug Administration) approval of the drug might affect the company's share price. Antonio, however, was eager to find out more about the drug as a possible treatment for his own Parkinson's disease. Antonio had first developed a resting tremor and been diagnosed with PD three years ago, when he was fifty-nine. He continued to work as an engineer and had already done a fair amount of library research on Parkinson's disease. He was concerned about how the disease would affect his retirement plans. He and his wife of thirty years, Diana, had planned that he would retire at sixty-five. They would then travel to southern Europe and north Africa. These plans depended, of course, on both good physical health and a financially sound 401K plan!*

Patients and families often ask doctors about drugs and other therapies being developed to treat Parkinson's disease—experimental compounds or experimental dosing schedules, for example. There are always new drugs and products "in the pipeline." It is important to remember that participation as a "subject" in a clinical trial helps society develop new medical treatments but does not guarantee any benefit to individual participants. The decision about whether to participate in a clinical trial should be made in consultation with the patient's health care team and appropriate family members.

Pharmaceutical companies, the National Institutes of Health (NIH), and others use clinical trials to test medications, treatments, or devices to determine which ones are safe and effective. The goal is to find which treatments work best for a carefully defined group of people. Participants, sometimes called study subjects, must meet strict criteria to enroll in any given study. A research coordinator and doctor at a university, doctor's office, or clinic typically evaluate a person's eligibility. There should be no fee to enroll in a clinical trial. In fact, subjects are sometimes paid for their participation. The National Institutes of Health fund many of the medical trials in the United States and even abroad. The NIH currently lists more than forty clinical studies in Parkinson's disease alone. Many involve experimental drug treatments.

This chapter describes the drug approval process and the methodology used in clinical research trials. Should you decide to participate in a clinical trial, you will find here questions to ask the researchers in order to understand the drug under investigation, the study itself, and what to expect. We also introduce some common medical terminology that will help you become a more educated consumer. Finally, we provide information to help interested readers find clinical research studies.

## The Long Road to Market

New drugs must be approved by the FDA before they can be offered for sale. Clinical trials are an integral part of the approval process. The FDA stipulates that drugs go through three phases of rigorous clinical testing. The three phases involve progressively larger numbers of people and testing over longer periods of time.

Phase 1 is to determine the metabolic and pharmacologic actions of the drug in humans and the side effects associated with increasing doses. The number of study subjects in a Phase 1 clinical trial is small. It varies with the drug but is usually between twenty and eighty people. Phase 2 is to determine the safety and effectiveness of the treatment. The number of study subjects is larger than in the first phase, generally anywhere from a few dozen to a few hundred participants. Finally, Phase 3 is to determine the long-term benefits of the medication, treatment, or device. A few hundred to a few thousand subjects may be enrolled in this phase.

## FDA History and the Drug Approval Process

In 1906 the FDA was given regulatory authority over the labeling and sale of drugs, but it was not until 1938 that Congress actually required drug manufacturers to obtain premarket approval from the FDA. In the second half of the twentieth century, a system of laboratory testing and human clinical trials was established to determine the safety and efficacy of drugs.

Evaluation of a potential drug begins in the laboratory. Before a drug can be tested in people, its physical and chemical properties must be analyzed in test tubes. The pharmacologic and toxic effects of the drug are then tested in animals. If these results show promise, the company developing the drug can apply to the FDA to begin testing in people. The application submitted to the FDA, known as the Investigational New Drug application (IND), must provide data from the experiments done in test tubes and in animals that justify testing the drug in humans. The IND must be reviewed and approved by the FDA before human clinical trials can begin.

Human clinical trials are conducted to find new safe and effective treatments for a particular disease. Before humans can be enrolled in a given clinical trial at a particular hospital, the institutional review board (IRB) of that hospital must also review and approve the details of the trial. The IRB is an independent body that includes physicians, nurses, and lay members of the community. Each hospital or clinic that participates in clinical trials must have its own IRB, whose job it is to review clinical research trials to ensure that they are run safely and fairly. The IRB is responsible for protecting the rights and welfare of subjects both before and during a clinical trial.

In Phase 1 clinical trials, a small number of healthy volunteers or patients are given the study drug. These studies assess the most common acute adverse effects and examine the size of the dose that people can take safely without a high incidence of side effects. If Phase 1 studies do not reveal significant problems, then the drug proceeds to Phase 2 testing.

In Phase 2 testing, the study drug is given to patients who have the condition that the drug is intended to treat. Researchers then assess whether the drug has a favorable effect on the condition. Up to several hundred patients are recruited for a Phase 2 trial. In a Phase 2 clinical research trial for a Parkinson's disease drug, for example, researchers would look for a statistically significant reduction in the UPDRS (United Parkinson's Disease Rating Scale, described in Chapter 2) score in people taking the experimental drug versus people who receive a placebo (an inactive substance that looks like the experimental drug). If results of Phase 2 studies are promising, then a large number of patients are recruited for Phase 3 trials.

Phase 3 testing is designed to assess safety, efficacy, and appropriate dosage of the study drug. Several hundred to several thousand patients participate. The patients are treated with either the study drug or a placebo, and are monitored for one to four years.

After Phase 3 trials are completed, a team of FDA physicians, statisticians, chemists, pharmacologists, and other scientists review the data. If this independent and unbiased review establishes that a drug's health benefits outweigh its known risks, the drug is approved for sale.

Although studies vary widely, clinical trials share some common characteristics. For example, participants may have to give frequent blood samples, take neuropsychological tests, or undergo frequent testing to assess their disease status. Participants may be asked to keep detailed records of their symptoms and to follow strict schedules. If you are interested in participating in a clinical trial, you should discuss the idea with your physician.

## What You Should Know Before Joining a Clinical Trial

Clinical trials expand our understanding of how a particular drug works and are fundamental to the process by which information obtained from laboratory work is applied in clinical practice. (See Figure 13.) It is very important to understand that volunteering for a clinical trial does not guarantee that you will receive the experimental drug. You may receive a placebo instead. Patients are randomized to receive one or the other. The patient will not know what he or she receives until the study is over. In most cases, neither will the doctor or staff.

The individual who participates in a clinical trial is not likely to benefit from his or her involvement. So why do it? Clinical trials are essential to the development of new drugs for the treatment of Parkinson's disease. Newer, more effective treatments will allow people with PD to lead full, active lives. By extending the number of years during which someone with Parkinson's disease can continue to work and live independently, society as a whole benefits. On a personal level, by helping in the development of new treatments for Parkinson's disease, you are in fact benefiting future generations.

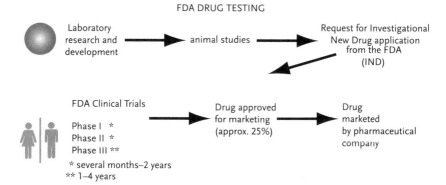

FIGURE 13.    Drug development. The steps involved in identifying compounds that may alleviate human disease are numerous and costly.
The initial steps take place in research laboratories and culminate in
the testing of compounds in animal models of human disease. Compounds that are not toxic to animals and have had some beneficial
effect are then reviewed by the FDA for human clinical trials. The results of the human trials are reviewed by the FDA at every step prior
to the approval of a specific drug for use in humans.

Possible complications of the treatment being tested are fully
explained by the people conducting the research trial, and patients must agree to all conditions. A member of the research
team explains why the study is being done and what the participant should expect. A consent form lays out the exact plan for
each step of the study, the side effects that may be experienced,
and how participation in the study may affect daily life. Should
you decide to participate in a clinical research trial, you will be
required to sign the consent form.

Here are a few questions to ask the research team, in order to
make an educated decision about joining a clinical trial:

- Why is this study being done?
- What kinds of tests and treatments are part of the study?

- How will the course of my Parkinson's disease be affected by the treatment?
- What other treatments can I get if I do *not* take part in the study?
- What are the possible short-term and long-term side effects of the study drug?
- How do risks and side effects of standard treatment compare with those of the study drug?
- How long will the study last?
- Will my insurance cover my participation in the study?
- If my insurance does not cover my participation, who or what institution is responsible for the costs?
- Will I have to stay in the hospital and, if so, how often and for how long during the course of this study?

Even after deciding to participate and signing the consent form, you can change your mind and stop your participation in a clinical trial at any time. If you decide to drop out of a clinical trial, speak to the study staff and discuss with them your reasons for doing so. This information may help in analyzing the data and in determining the safety, side effect profile, and ease-of-use of the medication or device that is being studied.

## Finding a Clinical Study

In February 2000, the U.S. government launched a website to provide health care professionals and the public with easy and accurate access to information about clinical trials. The website is called *ClinicalTrials.gov* and is a product of the 1997 FDA Modernization Act, which required an upgrade of many aspects of the FDA approval process. The developers of the site are the National Library of Medicine (NLM) of the National Institutes of Health and the FDA.

*ClinicalTrials.gov* is simple to use. The site can be searched by medical condition or by sponsor. The categories of sponsors—meaning funding agencies—include the NIH, other federal agencies, industries, universities, or any other type of public or private organization. Most of the studies take place in the United States and Canada, but some are overseas.

All totaled, *ClinicalTrials.gov* lists about 9,600 clinical studies. In December 2004, 132 of those studies were directly related to movement disorders and 79 were actively recruiting people with Parkinson's disease. The Parkinson's disease trials covered a broad range of topics, from uses of alternative treatment modalities, to mapping of dopamine receptors in the brain, to effects of experimental drugs on symptoms of Parkinson's disease and the dyskinesias that develop after long-term treatment with levodopa.

Strict criteria exist for determining whether someone is eligible to participate in a clinical trial, and *ClinicalTrials.gov* does a good job of summarizing the criteria for inclusion and exclusion, although the criteria are usually quite a bit more complex. Contact information is provided with each study so that patients and doctors can get in touch with the study coordinators directly. Another helpful feature of the site is that it links back to a site at the NIH that contains easy-to-understand information about Parkinson's disease.

There are other places to find listings of clinical research trials, too. One is PDTrials.org, a website begun in November 2004. It carries listings of clinical trials exclusively for Parkinson's disease. PDTrials.org was launched in partnership with the NIH and focuses on increasing participation in PD clinical trials. News updates about clinical trials are a standard feature of the site.

## Interpreting Medical Information

Reading information about a clinical trial may seem daunting. You are not alone if you feel confused and even intimidated when confronted by information about science and medicine. Even scientists sometimes have trouble understanding each other because of the specialized language and complexity of a specific scientific field that is not in their own area of expertise.

A good way to begin is to make a list of what you don't understand. Look up words and concepts in dictionaries, textbooks, and on the Internet. A medical dictionary is a good purchase. Try pronouncing new words; familiarity with different terms will make it easier to hold a conversation on the topic. Useful books and websites abound. Libraries are great resources not only for books but also for discovering links to helpful electronic resources. Parkinson's disease organizations can also answer many of your questions. Your own doctor and his or her staff should be willing to explain any elusive concepts.

Medical verbiage may read like a foreign language at first, but dissecting the information can make it manageable. Here is an example of seemingly difficult language, from a portion of an announcement telling people that a group of researchers is seeking patients to participate in a clinical trial:

> The University of Vermont College of Medicine in Burlington, Vermont, is calling for participants in a study entitled, "The Effects of Acute and Subchronic Nicotine on Attentional Functioning on Alzheimer's and Parkinson's Disease." The study will test whether varying dosages of intravenous nicotine, followed by nicotine administered by skin patch for two weeks, can improve attentional learning and motor impairments in Alzheimer's and Parkinson's disease patients. This short-term study aims to develop better treatments for patients with these diseases.

For many people, the new words in the paragraph would be *acute, subchronic, attentional functioning, intravenous, motor,* and *short-term*. A dictionary would tell you that *acute* means lasting a short time. Finding a definition for *subchronic* is harder and might require a search of the Internet and a little perseverance. *Subchronic,* according to guidelines provided by the International Organization for Standardization (ISO), means that exposure to the drug would be for a period of time less than 10 percent of the life span of the species tested. *Attentional functioning* is generally defined as you might expect, as an ability to pay attention. Neuropsychological tests determine different aspects of attention, like the ability to disregard irrelevant information or to remember a series of numbers or words. *Intravenous,* the dictionary reveals, means occurring within a vein or entering by way of a vein, and *motor* refers to movement. *Short-term* simply means for a short period of time.

Participating in clinical research is not for everyone, for medical and personal reasons. The best way to determine your medical eligibility and whether your temperament makes you a good candidate for a particular study is to ask plenty of questions so that the decision can be based on all the available facts.

# 12

# Communicating with Your Treatment Team

Now that you or your loved one has been diagnosed with Parkinson's disease, you will need to select a medical doctor to treat the condition and to help navigate the days, months, and years ahead. It is very important to choose a doctor with whom you feel comfortable because, in all likelihood, you will be getting to know that person and his or her medical staff very well.

You will have many new questions that only an experienced and trained professional can answer. If you worry about sounding petty, naïve, or even silly, we highly recommend that you abandon that fear. Select a doctor who truly believes that there is no such thing as a stupid question. Only then will you feel free to ask for the help you need.

You can begin the process of selecting a doctor by asking for recommendations from people and resources you respect. Here are some ideas:

- *Family physician.* Physicians know about the training and skill of their colleagues in the community.
- *Member of the clergy.* Most clergy members have knowledge based on their experience with other members of the congregation.
- *Local hospital.* Most hospitals have a physician on staff who treats patients with Parkinson's disease. Find out who that doctor is and be prepared to research the person's skills by

making inquiries to the state medical society, asking around, and interviewing the doctor in person. See below for important questions to ask of any potential doctor.

- *Parkinson's disease organization.* The National Parkinson Foundation (NPF), for example, provides an extensive list of physicians with special interest and skill in treating patients with Parkinson's disease. The list—complete with addresses, contact names, and phone numbers—is available on the NPF website (http://www.parkinson.org/index.htm) or by calling the organization toll free, at 1-800-327-4545.
- *Community meetings.* Many communities have disease-oriented patient and family groups that sponsor educational sessions and support groups. They are often organized by family members. There may be a Parkinson's disease support group in your community that meets on a regular basis. Most likely there will be many people in attendance willing to share their opinions about selecting a doctor.

## Selecting the Right Doctor for You

Research shows that the better the relationship between the patient, family, and doctor, the better the outcome for the patient. Many people are embarrassed to "interview" a doctor and staff, but we suggest it. The interview is not just about asking questions; it is also about observing and quietly evaluating what you have seen and heard.

True or false?

- It is important that I like the doctor.
- All members of the medical staff should be knowledgeable and understanding.
- My questions should be answered thoroughly and compassionately.

- The doctor should describe his or her philosophy concerning medical care of patients with Parkinson's disease.
- The doctor's waiting room should be accessible and comfortable.
- Even if I call frequently with pressing concerns, I should be treated with respect. My calls should be returned within a reasonable amount of time.

The answer to all these questions is *true*. It is important that you like and respect your doctor and that you feel at ease when you are in the office or discussing your concerns on the telephone. Ask yourself if this doctor is someone with whom you can work.

## A Specialist or a Primary Care Provider?

Depending on where you live, you may not have a choice about whether the doctor you select is a specialist in movement disorders (a neurologist with additional training in movement disorders) or a general neurologist. Both movement disorder neurologists and general neurologists have completed 3 years of intensive training in all neurological diseases. Movement disorder specialists have completed an additional 1–2 years of training specifically in movement disorders, and thus are highly skilled at the medical treatment of Parkinson's disease—though they probably have less daily experience in treating common neurological problems, such as headache! When you have a choice, it usually makes the most sense to see an expert in Parkinson's disease. Because of the varied symptoms and numerous medications used to treat Parkinson's disease, most people benefit by seeing a doctor who treats similar patients day in and day out.

Here's what many people do about their medical care, and

successfully. They depend on their primary care physician and a local, general neurologist for regular care, and then see a movement disorder neurologist about every six months. The specialist maintains contact with the local physicians through mail and phone correspondence. This way, patients have the benefit of a local doctor who is readily available and knowledgeable about the patient's overall medical condition plus an expert in Parkinson's disease who can fine-tune medications and serve as a consultant to both the primary care physician and the primary neurologist.

## Interviewing the Doctor and Office Staff

Remember that you have a right to ask questions about a doctor's skills, training, and style of work. You are entitled to obtain information about the medical practice that will provide your care. If the doctor were in your position, he or she would surely do the same.

Not everything has to be phrased as a question when you conduct the interview. Curiosity can sometimes be satisfied just by looking around. Obvious things to look for would be whether the office is clean, if phone calls are answered promptly, if the waiting room is comfortable and reading material is up-to-date, and if the wait to see the doctor is acceptable.

You will want to chat with the staff, too. Notice whether they are helpful and knowledgeable. Do they look happy? You might want to ask a question about Parkinson's disease on the basis of what you have read or heard. If you are answered respectfully and thoroughly, consider it a good sign. Mention that you are new to the practice and are wondering what to expect. You might be surprised by what you hear.

When it's time to see the doctor, look for a few niceties, such as a handshake and a comfortable chair for everyone. Notice whether the doctor is listening carefully and asking questions in a compassionate manner. Does he or she seem observant and attentive? If you are a family member, is the doctor including you in the conversation?

Doctors want their patients to be involved in their own care. That means asking questions in order to be well informed. The first meeting is a good place to begin. Here are some questions you can ask, to find out the doctor's experience with Parkinson's disease and its treatment:

- What percentage of your practice consists of people with Parkinson's disease?
- Have patients with Parkinson's disease always been part of your practice?
- What have you found is the best form of treatment for most patients?
- What would the treatment options be in our case?
- What is your availability at night and on weekends?
- Do your patients ever enroll in clinical trials?
- Could you tell us about laboratory or clinical research programs with which you are involved?
- Will your office be able to recommend a physical therapist, occupational therapist, speech therapist, or psychologist experienced in working with people with Parkinson's disease, if the need arises?

These questions should give you a good introduction to the doctor.

The doctor-patient relationship is a unique bond that varies depending on the people involved. It is important to feel comfortable with your doctor. Because Parkinson's disease is a chronic illness, you and your physician will be establishing a long-term relationship. You should be able to discuss the impact of Parkinson's disease on all aspects of your life.

## Always Be Prepared

Once you've chosen your doctor, be prepared to get the most out of every visit. If you see the doctor once every six months, you will surely have several observations to report and questions to ask. Unless they are written down, some are likely to be missed. Paradoxically, the things we forget are often the most important.

Keep a running list of questions and concerns. Before going into an appointment, ask yourself what you want to get out of the visit. You might even keep an alphabetical list of headings as a reminder:

Appetite
Bowel and bladder habits
Complementary and alternative medicine
Exercise
Gait
Illnesses (other)
Medications
Mood
Over-the-counter medicines
Sex
Sleep
Socializing
Stiffness
Swallowing
Travel
Voice
Weight
Work
Other

This list covers concerns about the person with Parkinson's disease. You might also include topics about family members and the impact of the disease on the patient's relationship with his or her loved ones.

Most doctors are pleased when their patients come to appointments prepared to talk and ask questions. It means that the patient is involved in his or her care. It also can save time in the appointment by bringing the biggest concerns to the surface right away. If you have been reading about Parkinson's disease, and you probably will be, use time during the appointment to ask questions about topics that are not clear or about which you want more information. Be respectful of the doctor's time by having the questions ready. If you find that they are not being answered or that you are dissatisfied for any other reason, you might want to think about whether this is the right doctor for you. Some offices employ a nurse who is skilled at answering questions from patients and families.

Thank the doctor and staff after each visit. Be sure to let them know that you appreciate their time and attention. They, like you, work hard and are glad to hear that they are making a difference.

## In Case of Emergency

You should ask your doctor about what to do in case of emergency, even though emergencies associated with Parkinson's disease are rare. Parkinson's disease is a chronic condition, so change does not happen suddenly and alarmingly. It occurs slowly, over months to years.

Families commonly think it's an emergency when they notice that the response to Parkinson's medications is not what it had been. Movements appear slower and more rigid. It is important to contact your doctor when this happens, but it is not an emergency. The doctor will make careful changes to the medication. Unlike the use of antibiotics for a bacterial infection such as pneumonia, medical treatment for Parkinson's disease requires a slow, careful adjustment in dosage and type of medicine used.

Also, do not be surprised if your symptoms of Parkinson's disease worsen if you have another illness, such as a cold or the flu. Although we do not know why this happens, it is common for an illness in another part of the body to aggravate the symptoms of Parkinson's disease. If this happens, it is important not to overreact and start adjusting the medications for Parkinson's disease. Although it may be difficult, wait for the symptoms of the acute illness to resolve. And remember, a worsening of a rest tremor or increased rigidity while someone is suffering from the flu does not mean that the course of the Parkinson's disease is getting worse.

# 13

# When Long-Term Arrangements Are Required

One of the most difficult decisions that families and patients face, and often try to avoid, is what to do if things become completely unmanageable. By this, in the extreme, we mean if the person with Parkinson's disease can no longer function independently or the family finds it impossible to meet the physical and emotional demands of the situation. Long-term arrangements in an extended-care or nursing facility can become necessary. It is best to address this early and frankly.

If you are the patient, face this possibility as soon as possible, think about it carefully, and make it clear to *all* family members, preferably in writing as well as verbally, how you want to live and die. By facing this challenging issue yourself, you are relieving family members of a tremendous burden. You might think of your leadership in the matter as a gift from you to them.

Unfortunately, when children are involved in making choices regarding extended-care or nursing home facilities for an ill parent, it is all too common for old rivalries and bad feelings to emerge and interfere with decision making. This tension is usually extremely upsetting for families already under a great deal of stress. It may be helpful to know that doctors see the same fears and anxieties in nearly every family they treat and that advanced planning can help avoid conflicts.

Here is a story that may have a familiar ring:

*Bill is seventy-five and has had Parkinson's disease for seventeen years. His wife, Sondra, is seventy-two and has bad arthritis. They live in the house where they raised their three children but only use the bottom floor because it's difficult for them both to climb the stairs.*

*Two of their children, Bill Jr. and Nancy, who is the youngest, live nearby. Their middle child, Roberta, lives 2,000 miles away and comes home for the Christmas holidays and for a week in the summer. Bill Jr. and Nancy alternate taking days off from work to go with their parents to their many doctor appointments. They manage other tasks, too. Nancy has arranged for lawn and housekeeping services for her parents, and Bill Jr. takes care of all the house repairs. Bill Jr. and Nancy have had some quiet, furtive discussions in which they talk vaguely about what to do if one or both parents become "really sick," but neither has brought up the subject of assisted living or nursing homes.*

*Bill Sr. and Sondra, whose own parents died at relatively young ages (all in their fifties), sometimes express disbelief that they have become as old as they are. They try to avoid discussions about the other's infirmities. They don't want to scare each other, and they continue, as they say, to "manage just fine."*

*Suddenly, though, Sondra has a massive stroke and ends up in the intensive care unit of a hospital. Bill Sr., Bill Jr., and Nancy maintain a constant vigil at the hospital and Roberta makes arrangements to fly home. She makes it to the hospital two days later.*

*Sondra survives, but it is clear to the physicians, nurses, and physical therapists who treat her that she will require constant nursing care. The social worker, discharge coordinator, nurses, and physicians at the hospital have periodic discussions with Bill Sr. and the rest of the family regarding the best arrangements for Sondra. Roberta is*

*quite shaken up and confides to her father and siblings that she be-
lieves they are all being pressured to get Mom out of the hospital.
She thinks that not everything that should have been done was done
to maximize Sondra's abilities. Her mom did not have high blood
pressure, she did not smoke, and there is no family history of stroke,
so how could this have happened? Why didn't her regular physician
pick up on some warning signs? And why is everyone giving up and
sending Mom to a nursing home?*

*After spending a week at Sondra's bedside, Roberta finally realizes
that her mom does, in fact, need constant care. She feels shocked
and confused, but Bill Jr. and Nancy are less upset because they understood their mother's needs almost immediately. They also know
that Bill Sr. is not healthy enough to care for Sondra. They want to
spare their dad from having to say, "I can't do it," so they begin to
look for a nursing home.*

*Although all three children are unhappy about having to put their
mom in a nursing facility, Bill Jr. and Nancy feel that it is the only
choice. Nancy goes on a tour of several homes that the hospital discharge coordinator has recommended; she and Bill Jr. also work out
a schedule whereby they and some cousins will drive Dad to the
home for daily visits. Roberta, by contrast, is horrified that her
brother and sister can make such plans. "Why not have Mom at
home, with an aide who comes in for a few hours every day? Dad
is not that sick," she says, "and they can still be together . . ."*

This is a common scenario, with some variations, of course,
in different families. The divisions between the children cause
significant tension and make it extremely difficult to come to
an agreement regarding the placement of their parent. In the
meantime, the hospital staff has completed its intensive treatment and evaluation of the patient. The insurance company is
eager to discharge the patient from the hospital, because she is
not getting any treatment there that could not be provided in a

skilled nursing facility. The hospital administration, fearing that the insurance company will refuse to pay for additional days in the hospital, is eager to see the family come to an agreement.

Help is available for resolving situations like this. The family described above—to avoid a growing disagreement that they feared could lead to a family feud—participated in a series of meetings with the hospital staff. Three times they talked with a hospital social worker and discharge planner. They each separately talked with the hospital chaplain, too. And the whole family met with the physicians, nurses, and therapists who treated Sondra. The emphasis was kept on what would be best for Sondra on the basis of the recommendations of the health care professionals who had no vested interest in the dynamics between the siblings or between them and their father. After these meetings, and after spending time talking together, all three children and their father finally agreed that Sondra would be best served in a nursing facility that was close to home. With the assistance of the discharge coordinator at the hospital, they found a good facility and transferred Sondra there.

There are several lessons to be learned from the experience of this family. One is how difficult it is to make a decision to change a living situation when decreasing health makes it necessary. Another is that even well-meaning and loving family members can complicate decision making because they may not fully understand the situation. Still another is that hospitals have trained staff to aid in resolving family conflict and facilitating decision making.

But perhaps the most important message is that it is far easier to think about and discuss assisted living and nursing home arrangements before they are needed.

We recommend that the Parkinson's disease patient and all the members of the family who could be faced with decisions about a living situation address the issue early and as often as necessary. You should look into the costs of an assisted-living facility. There are many types available, and the cost is substantial. Many have skilled nursing facilities with nurses available twenty-four hours a day. Some provide basic services and others are all-encompassing. A good resource for getting started is a publication from the National Institute on Aging called "Long-Term Care: Choosing the Right Place." Copies are available at www.niapublications.org/engagepages/longterm.asp.

Patients who make these decisions and have them in place should the need arise could save partners and family members from a difficult task at a time of extreme stress and anxiety. Families who do have to make the decision in a hurry because their loved one is hospitalized should remember that the professionals in the hospital are skilled at facilitating these discussions and at helping loved ones sort out their feelings. Although people often feel that they are the only ones to have ever gone through such a situation, they are not, and there are many people who can help.

## Choices

So what are the choices in living situations?

### Modifications to the Existing Home

Some health problems may simply require modifications to the patient's existing house. To minimize the risk of falls in the bathtub or shower stall, a grab bar can be added at minimal cost. In addition, the removal of area rugs will significantly reduce the risk of falls. By taking active steps to prevent injury, an individual can help ensure more time spent living independently in his or her own home. Below is a list of safety precautions that should be taken in the home after someone is diagnosed with

Parkinson's disease and before there are any falls or serious injury.

Evaluate the entrances into the home. If the Parkinson's patient must climb stairs to enter, install handrails on *both* sides of the steps. It does not matter how many steps there are—even one step is a fall risk.

Are there stairs within the home? If so, install a second handrail, if possible, so that your loved one can hold on to both sets of rails when climbing up or down the stairs. If the staircase is too wide, then consider installing an electric chair for moving between the first and second floor.

Area rugs are a significant fall hazard. Remove *all* area rugs and replace with wall-to-wall carpeting or maintain bare floors.

What about electrical cables? Are there lamps standing several feet from a wall, with a trail of cable going into the outlet? This is not safe. Rearrange furniture and change lighting schemes to avoid tripping hazards.

The bathroom is potentially the most dangerous room in the house. A towel rack is *not* a grab bar. A towel rack will hold the weight of two to three large towels, not the weight of an adult. Grab bars should be installed in the shower stall or tub, as well as in the wall of the bathroom, where the patient can reach while stepping out of the tub. Grab bars should be drilled into the wall stud itself, to ensure that they are strong enough to hold a person's weight. A shower chair in the tub will get around the difficulty with balance that those with Parkinson's disease have and minimize the risk of a fall in the tub or shower. And how about the toilet seat? The lower the seat, the more difficult it is to get up. You can install arms on either side of the toilet seat or replace the toilet seat itself. Home improvement stores carry a variety of bathroom fixtures that comply with the guidelines of the Americans with Disabilities Act (ADA) and are surprisingly stylish. (See Figure 14.)

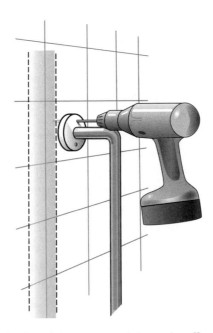

FIGURE 14.    Bathtub grab bar. For a grab bar to be effective, it must be drilled into the wall stud itself.

What about the bedroom? Typically, individuals get up once during the night to urinate. Are there nightlights to guide the way? Is it possible to hold on to a wall en route to the bathroom, or would a walker provide more support? If a walker and night-lights are not enough to allow safe travel from the bed to the bathroom, then consider using a bedside commode at night. The commode is placed close to the bed and should be cleaned out every morning so there is no residual smell of urine.

## In-Home Care

In-home care can vary from nonmedical assistance, to help with home upkeep, to private nursing care. Keep in mind that these services are not covered by an insurance plan, and so it is essential that you review your personal finances when making preparations. Examples of nonmedical care include landscaping services, house cleaning, laundry, and meal preparation. Examples of in-home medical care include visits by nurses to review medication regimens and ensure that there is no confusion between the doctor's instructions and what the individual is actually taking. For those who are unable to drive easily to their appointments, in-home physical therapy, occupational therapy, and nursing visits may be covered by insurance plans. However, the coverage provided for these services varies according to insurance plan and the patient's medical condition and needs. As part of the planning process, ask your insurance company which services are covered.

*Mohammed and Yasmin have been married for fifty-two years. Their two children are grown and live nearby with their own families. Mohammed is now eighty-two and is in relatively good health, taking only one medication to control his high blood pressure and an occasional aspirin or acetaminophen for minor aches and pains. Yasmin is seventy-five and was diagnosed with Parkinson's disease seven years ago. She is now slower in going about her daily activities, but she continues to perform all household tasks herself. Every week, she does the laundry and cleans the house. It takes her twice as long to complete these tasks as it has in the past. Both her children have urged her to get help at home, out of concern for her health and because they want her to rest, finally, after working so hard for so many years. Yasmin and Mohammed have resisted getting help at home out of fear that they would somehow be pushed into giving up their home and moving into a skilled nursing facility.*

*All of this changed, however, when Yasmin was hospitalized for pneumonia. She spent ten days in the hospital before returning home. Although she felt much better, Yasmin was still weak and not able to perform all the chores she had before her illness. While she was hospitalized, her children, with the help of the hospital social worker, were able to get her and Mohammed to agree to use a bi-weekly housekeeping service that would clean the house, do the laundry, and make dinner on the days they were working in the home. Fortunately, Yasmin and Mohammed had saved a significant amount of money and were able to afford these services without difficulty. Once they agreed to let "strangers" work in their home, it was relatively easy for them to agree to additional safety modifications as well. Their son, Hasan, was able to install a grab bar in every bathroom as well as a second handrail in the staircase that led from the first to the second floor. Hasan also installed handrails on the two steps leading from the garage into the kitchen.*

*Once Yasmin returned home and was feeling stronger, she and Mohammed decided to research assisted living facilities in their area. Although they were not yet ready to move, and did not need to, they decided to plan ahead and make arrangements to stay in a facility once they were unable to take care of a large home.*

## Assisted Living

Assisted living provides a combination of housing, personalized support services (like housekeeping or help with bathing), and health care for people who need help with activities of daily living but want to maintain privacy and independence. Activities of daily living are defined as the basic tasks of everyday life, such as eating, bathing, dressing, and toileting.

It is estimated that over one million Americans live in assisted-living residences. Accommodations are available for every income bracket. Some are run by nonprofit agencies and others are run by for-profit companies. Some are full service and others offer a limited menu, so to speak.

There is no single blueprint for the operation of an assisted-living residence. For more information, we recommend that you contact a national organization called the Assisted Living Federation of America (ALFA). ALFA has a website, www.alfa.org, where you can find information about services and lists of assisted-living residences in different areas of the country. It is a good idea to learn about the facilities in your area long before a member of your family might benefit from one, so that everyone will be prepared if the need arises.

*Helen had moved 150 miles to be near her son Tom. She lived in her own apartment, but she and Tom phoned each other and visited a few times a week. The symptoms of Helen's Parkinson's disease were mild at first but then problems with fine motor control began to interfere with her dressing and cooking. As concerns about her safety mounted, she and Tom decided it would be best if she moved to an assisted-living facility. There, she took her meals in a common dining room, got the help she needed, and otherwise lived independently. Safety was no longer a worry. Helen and Tom felt freer to enjoy their time together.*

### Skilled Nursing Facility

Skilled nursing facilities, commonly known as nursing homes, perform services such as administering medications, turning over patients in bed who cannot do it alone, or changing the dressings on wounds. In the United States, each state defines the type of care that may be administered only by a nursing home. To learn where the line between a skilled nursing facility and an assisted living facility is drawn in your state, see regulations at seniorresource.com.

Most people with Parkinson's disease and their families realize there may come a time when living at home under existing conditions is no longer safe for the PD patient or manageable for the family. Some household changes to reduce the risk of injury are easy, like putting a grab bar in the bathroom or replacing throw rugs with wall-to-wall carpeting. Other changes are extremely challenging, like bringing a health aide into the home or moving to a place where help is available on a part-time or full-time basis.

No one should underestimate the emotional, physical, and financial challenge involved when a family must make a major change in living arrangements owing to the need for long-term care. Families should strive to avoid conflict as much as possible by thinking about the possibility in advance and soliciting opinions from people who have a stake in decisions concerning the well-being of the person with PD. Recommendations from health care professionals and specially trained personnel should form the basis of family decisions.

# 14

# The Wedding

Special events like weddings and the arrival of grandchildren are joyous occasions that parents and children typically celebrate together. At such times we expect our loved ones, especially our parents, to be actively involved. But what happens if one parent has a chronic illness that makes it difficult for him or her to meet the family's expectations? The following story demonstrates how one family confronting Parkinson's disease worked together to solve this problem, and how they continue to face and meet new challenges.

## Monday, June 15: Five Days until the Wedding

Jennifer was busy with last-minute errands for her wedding. She had taken the previous week off from work and could hardly believe that she still had so many tasks on her to-do list. Fortunately, the final head count for the reception was in the hands of the caterer, and the band, photographer, and florist had all been confirmed.

Jennifer's fiancé, Rick, had picked up the wedding rings, been fitted for his tuxedo, and was recovering from the bachelor's party his friends had thrown for him the previous Friday night. Rick's remaining responsibilities were to attend the rehearsal and wrap up his Saturday morning round of golf with his groomsmen in time for everyone to shower, dress, and arrive at the wedding to welcome guests.

Jennifer, on the other hand, was still working on the seating arrangements for the reception. She wanted to make sure that everyone seated together had something in common. She also had to make sure that a few feuding relatives were seated at separate tables! More than anything else, however, Jennifer was nervous about walking down the aisle with her father. She was not nervous about herself; she was worried about her dad.

Dad was sixty-two, and eight years earlier he had been diagnosed with Parkinson's disease. He had a tremor and tended to walk with his head bent down. In the last few months, he would sometimes freeze while walking. Jennifer was afraid that her father would not make it down the aisle with her because he would either stumble, freeze, or fall. His symptoms intensified when he was nervous, and Jennifer knew that at her wedding they would both be nervous, happy, and sad all at once. Jennifer was afraid for her dad, afraid that he would fall in front of all their family and friends and be terribly embarrassed. Although she was ashamed to admit it, she was afraid that she would also be embarrassed if he fell, and angry because it would spoil the day.

Unbeknownst to Jennifer, her dad had been worrying, too. He wanted to walk his daughter down the aisle—safely and proudly. So about a month before the wedding, he made a smart move. He called his neurologist, explained the problem, and was immediately referred for physical therapy.

The physical therapist helped Jennifer's dad strengthen his leg muscles and practice consciously putting each foot completely down with every step. The therapist also recommended that Jennifer place twenty-four-inch-long pieces of tape at twelve-inch intervals on the white runner that would extend down the

center aisle of the chapel. This would serve as a concrete reminder to her dad of where each footstep should fall.

## Tuesday, June 16: Four Days before the Wedding

Jennifer and her mom and dad stretched the runner out as far as
it would go and put down the tape. They decided not to practice
on the runner just yet because they didn't want to soil it.

## Friday, June 19: Evening before the Wedding

At the rehearsal, Jennifer and her dad stand in the vestibule of
the church, out of sight of the guests, and practice walking.
Jennifer sets a metronome (another suggestion from the physical therapist) to help her dad get started and then walk at a regular and steady pace. They practice several times until they are
both comfortable and confident. Jennifer had chosen a wedding
gown without a train for two reasons: she preferred a simple
dress and it would be easier on her dad.

   Jennifer and her dad were also worried that he might not be
able to dance with her at the reception, with all the guests' eyes
on them and the photographer and videographer recording every moment. Again following the suggestion of the physical
therapist, Jennifer chose a slow song with a prominent beat for
her dance with her dad. Not only had Jennifer attended dance
class with her fiancé in the months before the wedding, but she
also brought Dad along a couple of times to work with her instructor, who had taught others with Parkinson's disease.

## Saturday, June 20: Wedding Day!

Jennifer is nervous, happy, and scared all at the same time.
While she dressed, and then as she posed for pictures, she

thought about how foolish she had been to worry about whether she should marry, ever.

Rick had to ask her twice! They had been dating for three years, and Rick said he had no doubt that she was the right woman for him. Although Jennifer loved him, she was worried that she might not be able to be a good wife and life partner—both her father and her maternal grandfather had been diagnosed with Parkinson's disease, and she thought the same might happen to her or their children. Her maternal grandfather had been diagnosed with Parkinson's disease in his seventies, and had died of lung cancer two years later. Although Jennifer was a child at the time, she remembered watching him shuffle around the garden with his hand shaking uncontrollably. After her dad's diagnosis, Jennifer had decided not to have children out of fear that, given the family history, her children would be at high risk for developing PD. She didn't discuss this issue with Rick until the first time he asked her to marry him. She hadn't discussed it with anyone before, not even her physician or her dad's neurologist.

After a long and difficult discussion, Rick finally convinced Jennifer to talk to her doctor, who then sent her to meet with a genetic counselor. After the physician and counselor explained that the vast majority of cases of Parkinson's disease are clearly not inherited, and reviewed what is understood about Parkinson's disease, Jennifer realized that she should go on and live life to the fullest without worrying about developing or passing along the disease. So when Rick proposed again, Jennifer said, "yes."

The wedding processional began, Dad and Jennifer walked down the aisle flawlessly, and the day was a huge success.


## Three Years Later

A few years after the wedding, Jennifer gives birth to her first child, Dylan. Dylan is the first grandchild on both sides of the family, and many relatives are eager to hold him. When Dylan is six weeks old, Rick's parents volunteer to baby-sit so Jennifer and Rick can go to a party. When Dylan is six months old, he spends the night with his paternal grandparents again, while Jennifer and Rick go on an overnight ski trip. Dylan loves spending time with all his grandparents.

Dylan begins to walk at one year and is running by the time he is two. Jennifer and Rick make plans to go away for a weekend and assume that Rick's parents will baby-sit again. But Jennifer's parents, particularly her dad, are eager to baby-sit and indulge their grandson.

In the five years since their wedding, the symptoms of Dad's Parkinson's disease have slowly worsened. He takes more medication and occasionally becomes frozen. A month ago, he fell down the two steps leading from the kitchen door to the garage. He and Jennifer's mom finally followed the advice of his neurologist and physical therapist and removed all the area rugs from their house. They also installed handrails for the steps leading from the kitchen door into the garage. As additional safety measures, they had a second handrail installed along the inside staircase and put a grab bar in the shower.

Jennifer is worried about leaving Dylan with her parents, because she does not think that her dad is well enough to chase after the baby. And she feels that her mom has enough to do just taking care of her dad. Her parents, however, do not see Dylan as much as they would like and are eager to spend more time with him.

Fortunately, Rick's parents and Jennifer's parents have become friendly and live within twenty miles of each other. Jennifer makes plans to leave Dylan with her parents, knowing that Rick's mom and dad are also keeping that weekend free and would be happy to help, even if it means stopping by to spend a few hours with Dylan at his maternal grandparents' home, or taking complete care of Dylan should something happen to Jennifer's dad. This solution worked for everyone and shows how, with creative thinking and a willingness to adjust as the situation demands, Parkinson's disease need not deprive patients or their families of the things they love most.

APPENDIX

NOTES

GLOSSARY

REFERENCES

INDEX

# Resources

Families coping with Parkinson's disease never need to feel that they are alone in the world. Organizations and individuals worldwide publish books, host websites, produce newsletters, and answer telephone calls, all about living and coping with Parkinson's disease. We hope that this book has answered many questions. But, as with any other disorder, the vast array of information about Parkinson's disease is constantly being updated with findings and facts that individuals and families might find useful for their own circumstances.

Our advice is to stay informed. Continue to ask questions. Work hard to maintain a high quality of life. Although living with a chronic disease like Parkinson's can be difficult, there are many opportunities for feeling good, and lots of people who can help you discover ways to make life easier or more enjoyable.

Some of the resources in this list are geared toward scientists, physicians, and other professionals. The information may be about the pathophysiology of neuron loss in Parkinson's disease, for example, a challenging topic even for scientists who work in the field. Choose the resources that are the best fit for your level of interest and knowledge.

We believe that the resources we provide here are among the best. The short description that accompanies each resource is meant as an overview of how that agency or website might provide you with some useful insight or tangible help. We find the information that comes from U.S. government organizations and from professional Parkinson's disease foundations especially well researched. Many other resources, such as hospital websites, for example, base their articles and facts on government reports, so you can save time by going to the original source.

A few words of caution: Avoid advice that sounds unrealistic or questionable. Your physician is the best resource when you have concerns about information received outside his or her office. Your health and well-being are at stake, so move with care through the abundance of information that is available. Much of it is solid, but some is truly spurious and even inaccurate or harmful.

Note that website addresses, phone numbers, addresses, other contact information, and even content are subject to change. We can only guarantee that the information provided here was accurate at the time this book was published. We encourage you to persevere in finding the information that will make you better prepared for whatever is to come.

## PROFESSIONAL SOCIETIES

### American Academy of Neurology (www.aan.com)
1080 Montreal Ave.
Saint Paul, MN 55116
Tel: (800) 879-1960 or (651) 695-2717

The AAN is a professional society for medical specialists. The stated mission of the AAN is to advance the art and science of neurology, and thereby promote the best possible care for patients with neurological disorders. AAN offers professional development, career enhancement, and practice-improvement opportunities for physicians and other health care providers. The AAN website contains a brief section for the public, with links to other websites dedicated to neurological diseases.

### American Neurological Association (www.aneuroa.org)
5841 Cedar Lake Rd., Suite 204
Minneapolis, MN 55416
Tel: (952) 545-6284

The ANA is a professional society of academic neurologists and neuroscientists. The society's mission is to advance the goals of academic neurology, train and educate neurologists and other physicians in the neurological sciences, and expand the understanding of diseases of the nervous system and their treatment.

## U.S. GOVERNMENT AGENCIES AND WEBSITES

### ClinicalTrials.gov (www.clinicaltrials.gov)

Many patients and families ask about research in Parkinson's disease, hoping to participate in what is called clinical research or a clinical trial. The website ClinicalTrials.gov lists ongoing research trials, federally and privately funded, and provides information about the purpose of the research, criteria for participation, and contact information. At times, there are forty or more studies listed under the heading of Parkinson's disease. Before joining any trial, speak with your personal physician. Given the sheer number of research trials, it is difficult for one doctor to keep up with all the research being done, and your diligence might reveal a study that could be appropriate for you.

### Healthfinder (www.healthfinder.gov)

Healthfinder is an extensive and useful website. It contains health news, information about health care resources, and a library rich with information about health and medicine. Information about Parkinson's disease ranges from general (overviews, descriptions of the disease) to quite specialized (depression and Parkinson's disease, occupational therapy, and more). The healthfinder project is coordinated by the Office of Disease Prevention and Health Promotion (ODPHP).

### MEDLINEplus (www.medlineplus.gov)

This website is another authoritative and valuable health-information resource sponsored by the United States government. The site is updated daily in English and Spanish. It is geared toward both health professionals and consumers, and provides facts and findings about more than six hundred conditions. For Parkinson's disease, it reports the latest news and contains information about clinical and laboratory research, disease management, medications, nutrition, treatments, genetics, and legal matters. On February 6, 2003, for example, the site posted a report that Medicare would cover the cost of deep-brain stimulation for essential tremor and Parkinson's disease. The Parkinson's disease section of MEDLINEplus can be accessed at www.nlm.nih.gov/medlineplus/parkinsonsdisease.html.

## National Center for Complementary and Alternative Medicine (www.nccam.nih.gov)
NCCAM Clearinghouse
P.O. Box 7923
Gaithersburg, MD 20898
Tel: (888) 644-6226

NCCAM is part of the National Institutes of Health. The center supports research on complementary and alternative medicine and distributes information and advisories about CAM treatments. One recent clinical trial funded by NCCAM examines the effect of Chinese exercise modalities on physical fitness and motor control. Another tests magnetic brain stimulation in patients with Parkinson's disease and severe depression.

## National Institute of Neurological Disorders and Stroke (www.ninds.nih.gov)
NIH Neurological Institute
P.O. Box 5801
Bethesda, MD 20824
Tel: (800) 352-9424 or (301) 496-5751
TTY (for people using adaptive equipment): (301) 468-5981

Like NCCAM, NINDS is part of the National Institutes of Health. NINDS funds research into a broad array of neurological disorders, including Parkinson's disease. Studies in Parkinson's disease are aimed at discovering causes, finding better treatments, preventing the disease, and even finding a cure. A special section of the NINDS website describes the goal for Parkinson's disease research, which is to "ensure that extraordinary opportunities to move toward a cure are adequately supported and that critical obstacles to progress are addressed."

The website of NINDS contains valuable, up-to-the-minute facts and information about research findings and treatments for Parkinson's disease. It links to the government website ClinicalTrials.gov, which provides information on research studies that are currently recruiting subjects.

## PDTrials.org (www.PDtrials.org)

This website was developed as part of a campaign (Advancing Parkinson's Therapy Campaign, or APT) to increase patient participation in clinical trials. The site includes listings of clinical trials exclusively for Parkinson's disease and also regulatory news updates of interest to PD patients. APT is led by the Parkinson's Disease Foundation in collaboration with other PD advocacy groups and in partnership with the National Institutes of Health.

### PARKINSON'S DISEASE ORGANIZATIONS

## American Parkinson Disease Association
## (www.apda@apdaparkinson.org)
1250 Hylan Blvd., Suite 4B
Staten Island, NY 10305-1946
Tel: (800) 223-2732 or (718) 981-8001; Calif.: (800) 908-2732

The national office of the APDA coordinates the operations of sixty-five chapters across the United States and hundreds of support groups. The APDA helps people with Parkinson's disease and their families by providing education, referrals to medical care, and counseling. It is also a funding source for research on the causes and treatment of Parkinson's disease.

## Michael J. Fox Foundation for Parkinson's Research
## (www.michaeljfox.org)
Grand Central Station
P.O. Box 4777
New York, NY 10163
Tel: (212) 213-3525

The MJFF provides funding for research into causes and cures for Parkinson's disease. A mission of the foundation is to increase the pace of discovery by supporting innovative research.

MJFF has partnered with the Parkinson's Disease Foundation,

National Parkinson Foundation, Parkinson Alliance, other private funders, and the National Institutes of Health to support a "fast-track" research initiative designed to fund novel research proposals.

### Movement Disorder Society (www.movementdisorders.org)
611 East Wells St.
Milwaukee, WI 53202
Tel: (414) 276-2145

The MDS is an international professional society of clinicians and scientists who are interested in Parkinson's disease and other movement disorders. The mission of the MDS is to advance the neurological sciences pertaining to movement disorders by providing educational programs for clinicians, scientists, and the general public and promoting research into causes, prevention, and treatment of the various movement disorders.

### National Parkinson Foundation (www.parkinson.org)
1501 N.W. 9th Ave.
Bob Hope Research Center
Miami, FL 33136-1494
mailbox@parkinson.org
Tel: (800) 327-4545 or (305) 243-6666; Fla.: (800) 433-7022

The goal of NPF is—through research support—to find the cause of Parkinson's disease and a cure. Education of patients, caregivers, and the public is also part of the NPF mission through support groups, seminars, and publications.

### Parkinson Alliance (www.parkinsonalliance.net)
211 College Rd. East
Princeton, NJ 08540
admin@parkinsonalliance.net
Tel: (800) 579-8440 or (609) 688-0870

The Parkinson Alliance raises money for pilot research projects that allow researchers to qualify for major funding from the National Institute of Neurological Disorders and Stroke of the National Institutes of Health. The alliance is a nonprofit organization that, because of a relationship with the Tuchman Foundation, is able to channel 100 percent of the funds it raises into research. The Tuchman Foundation was formed to raise funds from corporations, associations, and individuals throughout the country. The funds raised go to a variety of causes—most notably to support research to find a cure for Parkinson's disease.

**Parkinson's Action Network (www.parkinsonsaction.org)**
300 N. Lee St.
Alexandria, VA 22314
Tel: (800) 850-4726 or (703) 518-8877; Calif.: (707) 544-1994

PAN is a patient-advocacy group working to increase federal support of research on Parkinson's disease. The group advocates for increased investment of public monies and an accelerated pace of research and new product approval. PAN also works to ensure patient access to existing and experimental treatments and to prevent discrimination in the workplaces of people with Parkinson's disease.

**Parkinson's Disease Foundation (www.parkinsons-foundation.org)**
710 West 168th St.
New York, NY 10032-9982
info@pdf.org
Tel: (212) 923-4700 or (800) 457-6676

The PDF seeks to help people with Parkinson's disease and their families by providing information, sponsoring professional and community conferences, awarding research grants and training fellowships, and advocating for increased spending by the federal government on research into the causes of Parkinson's disease and a cure.

**Parkinson's Institute (www.parkinsonsinstitute.org)**
1170 Morse Ave.
Sunnyvale, CA 94089-1605
Tel: (800) 786-2958 or (408) 734-2800

The roots of the Parkinson's Institute were in the discovery that the drug MPTP (1-methyl, 4-phenyl, 1,2,3,6-tetrahydropyridine) could be used to create Parkinson-like symptoms in experimental animals, a significant advance for the research community. The finding was an unfortunate outcome of illicit drug use by individuals in California who took a street drug contaminated with MPTP; they developed a movement disorder much like Parkinson's disease. The focus of the Parkinson's Institute is threefold: patient care, clinical research, and basic research.

### Parkinson Society Canada (www.parkinson.ca)
4211 Yonge St., Suite 316
Toronto, Ontario M2P 2A9
Tel: (800) 565-3000 or (416) 227-9700

The Parkinson Society of Canada considers itself the national voice for Canadians living with Parkinson's disease. Its purpose is to ease the burden for people with Parkinson's disease and for their care-givers and to raise money to find a cure. The Parkinson Society of Canada publishes helpful materials, sponsors conferences, and provides various additional means of support. The society has partner organizations throughout Canada.

### Worldwide Education and Awareness for Movement Disorders (www.wemove.org)
204 West 84th St.
New York, NY 10024
Tel: (800) 437-MOV2

The organization known as the Worldwide Education and Awareness for Movement Disorders (WE MOVE) calls itself "the Internet's most comprehensive resource for movement disorder information," and it is certainly rich and useful. It provides valuable information for patients, families, and health care professionals. The mission of WE MOVE is to increase knowledge and promote timely diagnosis and treatment in order to improve quality of life for people with movement disorders.

### Travel Access (www.access-able.com)

Before planning a trip, find out what services are available at your destination and how accessible tourist sites and hotels are in various parts of the world. The internet site www.access-able.com provides information regarding personal travel experiences to different cities, all over the world, as well as a list of travel agents who specialize in helping those with special needs.

### Visiting Nurses Association of America (www.vnaa.org)

The VNAA is the national association of nonprofit, community-based home health organizations known as Visiting Nurse Associations (VNAs). VNAs share a mission to bring compassionate, high-quality, and cost-effective home care to individuals in their respective communities. To find out what in-home health care services are available in your community, go to the website listed above or find your local VNA in the yellow pages.

# Notes

## 1. WHAT IS PARKINSON'S DISEASE?

1. See: www.cdc.gov/nchs/releases/03news/lifeex.htm.

## 3. RISK FACTORS

1. A. Paganini-Hill, "Risk Factors for Parkinson's Disease: The Leisure World Cohort Study," *Neuroepidemiology,* 20 (2001): 118–124.

## 4. TREATMENT

1. The authors would like to thank Mara Wernick-Robinson, a physical therapist in the Department of Physical Therapy at Massachusetts General Hospital, and Suzanne Danforth, a speech therapist in the Department of Speech Therapy at Massachusetts General Hospital, for their help in preparing this chapter.

## 8. DEPRESSION

1. "Cognitive and Emotional Aspects of Parkinson's Disease," National Institute of Neurological Disorders and Stroke, National Institute on Aging, and National Institute of Mental Health working group meeting (January 24–25, 2001), unpublished summary.

2. M. A. Mensal, D. E. Robertson-Hoffman, and A. S. Bonapace, "Parkinson's Disease and Anxiety: Comorbidity with Depression," *Biological Psychiatry,* 34 (1993): 465–470.

3. A. G. Schuurman et al., "Increased Risk of Parkinson's Disease after

Depression: A Retrospective Cohort Study," *Neurology*, 58 (2002): 1501–1504.

## 9. DEMENTIA

1. T. Foltynie et al., "The Cognitive Ability of an Incident Cohort of Parkinson's Patients in the UK: The Campaign Study," *Brain*, 127 (2004): 550–560.

2. G. Levy et al., "Combined Effect of Age and Severity on Risk of Dementia in Parkinson's Disease," *Annals of Neurology*, 51 (2002): 722–729.

3. M. T. Hu et al., "Cortical Dysfunction in Non-Demented Parkinson's Disease Patients: A Combined (31)P-MRS and (18)FDG-PET Study," *Brain*, 123 (2000): 340–352.

## 10. ALTERNATIVE THERAPIES

1. M. Angell and J. P. Kassirer, "Alternative Medicine: The Risks of Untested and Unregulated Remedies," *New England Journal of Medicine*, 328 (1998): 839–841.

2. P. R. Rajendran, R. E. Thompson, and S. G. Reich, "The Use of Alternative Therapies by Patients with Parkinson's Disease," *Neurology*, 57 (2001): 790–794.

3. http://nccam.nih.gov/

4. C. Shults et al., "Effects of Coenzyme $Q_{10}$ in Early Parkinson Disease: Evidence of Slowing of the Functional Decline," *Archives of Neurology*, 59 (2002): 1541–1550.

5. www.amtamassage.org; last accessed October 11, 2002.

6. S. L. Wolf et al., "Reducing Frailty and Falls in Older Persons: An Investigation of Tai Chi and Computerized Balance Training," Atlanta FICSIT Group, Frailty and Injuries: Cooperative Studies of Intervention Techniques, *Journal of the American Geriatric Society*, 44 (1996): 489–497.

# Glossary

**Acetylcholine**   A chemical neurotransmitter that is released from the ends of nerve fibers. Acetylcholine is involved in the regulation of essential functions of the body, such as heart rate and respiratory rate.

**Activities of daily living (ADL)**   Basic tasks of everyday life, such as eating, bathing, dressing, toileting, and transferring from bed to chair or chair to an upright position.

**Akathisia**   A feeling of restlessness and the urge to move. Akathisia is a side effect of some antidepressant and antipsychotic medications and can be quite distressing.

**Akinesia**   A neurological term for lack of movement.

**Amino acids**   The chemical "building blocks" of proteins.

**Anhedonia**   Inability to derive pleasure from normally pleasurable acts. Anhedonia can be a symptom of depression.

**Anticholinergic**   A medication that opposes or blocks the action of acetylcholine. Two examples of anticholinergic drugs are trihexyphenidyl (Artane) and benztropine (Cogentin).

**Anxiety**   A heightened state of concern. A person who is anxious might feel nervous or have a sinking feeling that something has gone terribly wrong.

**Apathy**   A lack of emotion or feeling; indifference.

**Aphasia**   An impairment of the ability to use or understand words.

**Aspiration**   Inhalation of food or liquid into the airways or lungs, rather than into the stomach. Aspiration can result in pneumonia.

**Ataxia**   A loss of balance caused by a failure of the brain to coordinate movement. People who are ataxic appear wobbly and uncoordinated.

**Blepharospasm**   Uncontrolled contraction of muscles of the face surrounding the eye. The eyelids close and can be hard to open naturally.

**Bradykinesia**   A neurological condition, referring to slowness of movement. Bradykinesia is one of the cardinal signs of Parkinson's disease.

**Bradyphrenia**   A neurological condition, referring to slowness of thought processes.

**Cachexia**   A state of malnutrition.

**Carbidopa**   A drug that is administered along with levodopa (L-dopa) to prevent the L-dopa from being metabolized ("used up") before it enters the brain.

**Cardinal signs**   The most common signs exhibited by a majority of people with a disorder. Parkinson's disease is diagnosed through the appearance of cardinal signs in a patient.

**Cognition**   Mental processes, including all thinking and information processing. Cognition includes activities like using language and arithmetic during a trip to the grocery store, complex decision making like selecting between two job offers, and the ability to understand things from another person's perspective.

**Constipation**   Infrequent bowel movements, or the passing of hard stools, or straining to have a bowel movement. In people with Parkinson's disease, constipation occurs because the muscle of the colon contracts too slowly, causing the stool to move through it too slowly.

**Deep-brain stimulation**   A technique in which an electrode is implanted in the patient's brain to control symptoms of Parkinson's disease. (See Globus pallidus for details.)

**Delusion**   A false belief. In Parkinson's disease, the development of delusions can be related to medications in some patients. For example, an American's belief that he is the King of England is a grandiose delusion. Other kinds of delusions include delusions of paranoia (of malicious plots) and somatic delusions (of illness).

**Dementia**   A progressive and irreversible decline in a person's ability to form new memories, retrieve old memories, and perform complex tasks.

**Depression**   Excessive sadness characterized by persistently low mood or significant loss of pleasure and interest. Depression is a common psychological event in Parkinson's disease. It can usually be treated successfully with antidepressant medications.

**Diuretic**   A drug or other substance (e.g., coffee) that increases the production of urine.

**Dopamine**   A chemical neurotransmitter that is released at the ends of nerve fibers. Dopamine is essential for the proper functioning of the brain. People with Parkinson's disease do not have enough dopamine in their brains.

**Dopamine agonist**   A drug that works by binding to receptors on cells to trigger the same response as dopamine.

**Drug "holiday"**   A brief period of time when a prescribed medicine that is normally taken on a daily basis is not taken. People sometimes take a drug holiday to reduce side effects of medicines.

**Dysarthria**   An abnormality of speech due to impairment of the tongue or other muscles of the head and neck that are essential for speaking.

**Dyskinesia**   Excessive movement of muscles in the face or limbs that cannot be controlled voluntarily. Dyskinesias are a common side effect of levodopa (L-dopa) therapy for Parkinson's disease.

**Dysphagia**   Difficulty swallowing, or the inability to swallow.

**Dysthymia**   A mild, chronic form of depression that is characterized by low energy, decreased self-esteem, sad mood, and tearful episodes.

**Dystonia**   An involuntary muscle spasm that causes an abnormal posture. The most common site for dystonia in Parkinson's disease is the foot.

**Edema**   Swelling caused by the excessive accumulation of fluid in tissues.

**Essential tremor**   Tremor that occurs when a part of the body is in motion or held in a particular position. Essential tremor is the most common type of tremor, occurring most commonly in the hands, forearms, and head; the legs and torso are rarely involved. Essential tremor can be confused with the tremor of Parkinson's disease.

**Executive function**   A person's ability to plan and perform complicated tasks.

**Festination**   Walking with short, quick, shuffling steps. Festination is common in Parkinson's disease.

**Free radicals**   Molecules formed constantly as the body breaks down food, repairs injuries, maintains normal metabolism, and so forth. Free radicals are highly biologically reactive and have the potential to cause damage to body tissues.

**Gait disorder**   A slowing of gait speed, lack of accuracy, or lack of smooth or symmetric body movement while walking.

**Gene**   A functional section of genetic material, composed of DNA molecules, that is a portion of a chromosome, located in the nucleus of every cell. A gene instructs cells to make a particular protein.

**Globus pallidus**   An area of the basal ganglia in the brain. Experimental evidence suggests that the globus pallidus is overactive in people with Parkinson's disease; as a result, it sends strong inhibitory messages to the motor cortex of the brain, which causes the symptoms of Parkinson's disease. It is the target site for the surgical treatment pallidotomy, and one of the sites for deep-brain stimulation.

**Hallucination**   A false perception that occurs without any external sensory stimulation. Visual hallucinations described by people with Parkinson's disease are usually a side effect of Parkinson medications.

**Hoehn and Yahr Scale**   A standard scale for rating mobility commonly used by physicians to evaluate a person's disability from Parkinson's disease.

**Hypersexuality**   Unusual or excessive concern with, or indulgence in, sexual activity.

**Hypokinesia**   Decreased, diminished, or slow motor movement in response to a stimulus.

**Hypomimia**   Decreased facial expression. In Parkinson's disease, the loss of facial expression can be slight, as in a "poker face," or completely absent.

**Hypophonia**   A weak, soft voice. In Parkinson's disease, hypophonia is caused by the fact that the movements of the palate and the back of the throat, which help in generating a loud voice, are not working as quickly as they should. The Lee Silverman Voice Treatment (LSVT) method is sometimes used in Parkinson's patients to raise voice volume.

**Levodopa (L-dopa)**   A drug that replaces the dopamine that is missing from the brains of people with Parkinson's disease. Levodopa is a natural precursor to dopamine and is given in combination with another medication, carbidopa. Levodopa is most effective in reducing tremor, rigidity, and akinesia.

**Metabolism**   The basic chemical process that occurs in every cell in every living thing to produce energy. Metabolism is essential for life.

**Micrographia**   Small handwriting. In Parkinson's disease, handwriting becomes smaller and more cramped because of the inability to control fine motor movements.

**Mitochondria**   Tiny structures inside cells where the energy needed for each cell to survive is produced.

**Motor fluctuations**   A failure of L-dopa to provide a predictable effect on motor symptoms after long-term use of the drug. The reason for motor fluctuations is poorly understood.

**MPTP**   A drug (N-methyl-4-phenyl-1,2,3,6-tetrahydropyridine) that causes Parkinson-like symptoms. It was created by illicit drug makers, who thought they had made a version of a narcotic drug. MPTP is now employed as a tool in research on Parkinson's disease.

**Multiple system atrophy (MSA)**   A neurodegenerative disease marked by a combination of symptoms affecting movement, blood pressure, and other body functions. Multiple System Atrophy is sometimes confused with Parkinson's disease. (See also Parkinson plus syndrome.)

**Neuron**   A cell of the nervous system. There are many different types of neurons, with different functions and in different locations of the brain, spinal cord, and in other places in the body.

**Neurotransmitter**   A chemical that is released from the end of a neuron. It signals an adjacent nerve or tissue to increase or decrease its activity.

**"Off" period**   A period of time when a medication intended to control Parkinson's symptoms does not work.

**"On" period**   A period of time when benefit is derived from a medication, and disability from Parkinson's symptoms is lessened.

**Parkinson plus syndrome**   Several Parkinson-like neurodegenerative disorders. The doctor must consider these other conditions when making a diagnosis of Parkinson's disease. Multiple system atrophy (MSA) and progressive supranuclear palsy (PSP) are two examples of Parkinson plus disorders.

**Parkinson's disease**   A progressive disease caused by a deficiency of dopamine in the brain. A set of three (or four) cardinal signs are diagnostic of Parkinson's disease. No two Parkinson's patients progress at the same rate.

**PD**   A common abbreviation for Parkinson's disease.

**PET**   Abbreviation for positron emission tomography. PET is a noninvasive method to study metabolism—and identify metabolically active sites—within the brain and other organs.

**Placebo drug**   A preparation that has no specific pharmacological activity ("sugar pill"). A placebo is given to some participants (a control group) in a controlled clinical trial while other participants receive the experimental medication. Differences between outcomes of the two participant groups can be attributed to the effect of the experimental medication. The experimental medication must produce better results than the placebo to be considered effective.

**Pluripotent**   Cells that are pluripotent have the ability to develop into different kinds of cells found throughout the body.

**Progressive supranuclear palsy (PSP)**   A rare brain disorder that causes progressive difficulty with control of gait and balance. The most obvious sign of the disease is an inability to voluntarily move the eyes, which occurs because of lesions in the area of the brain that coordinates eye movements. PSP can be confused with Parkinson's disease. (See also Parkinson plus syndrome.)

**Protein**   A dietary compound consisting of amino acids that is essential for the growth and repair of tissues of the body.

**Psychosis**   A mental disorder characterized by the inability to think clearly, communicate rationally, interact appropriately, and generally understand the surrounding world. Symptoms can be extremely debilitating. Psychotic symptoms include delusions and hallucinations. Many people with a psychotic disorder get effective relief from antipsychotic medications. Psychotic symptoms can also develop as a side effect of medications used to treat Parkinson's disease.

**Rest tremor**   A tremor that occurs in a body part that is at rest but does not occur with voluntary movement. Rest tremor is characteristic of Parkinson's disease. (Contrast with Essential tremor, above.)

**Rigidity**   Increased stiffness in a muscle, perceived when the muscle is moved by someone else.

**Schwab and England Scale**   A daily living scale that evaluates a person's ability to live independently. It is scored in 10 percent increments: 100 percent indicates that a person is independent and able to do all chores without slowness, difficulty, or impairment; 0 percent indicates the person is unable to perform basic self-care tasks. The scale is commonly used to assess the abilities of Parkinson's patients.

**Sialorrhea**   Drooling. Drooling is quite common in several neurological diseases, including Parkinson's. There are several therapies that sometimes control sialorrhea, including injections of botulinum toxin (Botox) into one or more salivary glands.

**Side effect**   An undesired outcome of a medication or medical procedure.

**Sign**   Any objective evidence of an illness. Signs are definitive and independent of a patient's subjective impressions. (Contrast with Symptom.)

**SPECT**   Abbreviation for single photon emission computed tomography. SPECT is a noninvasive imaging procedure used to study blood flow in regions of the brain, and to study the attachment of neurotransmitters and dopamine agonists to dopamine receptors. This allows physicians to evaluate the extent of dopamine loss in people with PD.

**Substantia nigra**   A region of the basal ganglia of the brain. Cells of the substantia nigra are normally rich in dopamine, but in people with Parkinson's disease, substantia nigra cells die and the brain becomes deficient in dopamine.

**Symptom**   The subjective perception an individual has about a change in his or her body. Contrast Symptom with a Sign, which a doctor can see or measure.

**Tremor**   An involuntary movement of a part of the body caused by alternating contractions of opposing muscles. (See also Essential tremor and Rest tremor.)

**UPDRS**   Abbreviation for the United Parkinson's Disease Rating Scale, which is used to measure motor skills, cognitive (thinking) abilities, behavior (for example, activities of daily living), and other aspects of Parkinson's disease.

**Urinary incontinence**   An inability to retain urine.

**"Wearing off"**   The progressive shortening of the "on" (effective) period that follows a dose of L-dopa. Over time, most people, including friends and family, notice that L-dopa therapy works less well, and bradykinesia, tremor, and other symptoms reappear sooner between doses.

# References

We recommend selecting books and articles from this list as a way to expand your knowledge of Parkinson's disease. Medical and scientific articles are from professional journals and can nearly always be found in a medical library. Some articles are available over the Internet; often a small fee is charged for accessing the entire article, but a brief summary (an abstract) is usually free. Many public libraries subscribe to the more popular journals or are able to borrow them from other libraries.

## GENERAL INFORMATION

Calne, D. B. "Parkinsonism and Other Extrapyramidal Diseases." In D. A. Warrell et al., eds., *Oxford Textbook of Medicine,* vol. 3, 4th ed. Oxford: Oxford University Press, 2003, pp. 1053–1057.

Crucian, G. P., and M. S. Okun. "Visual-Spatial Ability in Parkinson's Disease." *Frontiers in Bioscience,* 1:8 (Sept. 1, 2003): S992–997. Review.

Duvoisin, R. C., and J. Sage. *Parkinson's Disease: A Guide for Patient and Family.* Philadelphia: Lippincott Williams and Wilkins, 2001.

Fox, M. J. *Lucky Man: A Memoir.* London: Ebury, 2002.

Gillingham, F. J., and M. C. Donaldson, eds. *Schwab and England Activities of Daily Living.* Third Symposium of Parkinson's Disease. Edinburgh, Scotland: E and S Livingstone, 1969, pp. 152–157.

Jankovic, J., and E. Tolosa, eds. *Parkinson's Disease and Movement Disorders*, 4th ed. Philadelphia: Lippincott Williams and Wilkins, 2002.

Kondracke, M. *Saving Milly: Love, Politics, and Parkinson's Disease.* New York: Perseus Books Group, 2001.

Nehlig, A. ed. *Coffee, Tea, Chocolate, and the Brain.* London: Taylor and Francis, 2004.

Sawada, H., and S. Shimohama. "Estrogens and Parkinson Disease: Novel Approach for Neuroprotection." *Endocrine*, 21:1 (June 2003): 77–79. Review.

Torpy, J. M., C. Lynm, and R. M. Glass. *Journal of the American Medical Association* patient page: Parkinson Disease. *Journal of the American Medical Association*, 291:3 (Jan. 21, 2004): 390.

William, J., et al. *Parkinson's Disease: A Complete Guide for Patients and Families.* Baltimore: Johns Hopkins University Press Health Book, 2003.

DIAGNOSIS

Tickle-Degnen, L., and K. D. Lyons. "Practitioners' Impressions of Patients with Parkinson's Disease: The Social Ecology of the Expressive Mask." *Social Science and Medicine*, 58:3 (Feb. 2004): 603–614.

CARE

Calne, S. M., and A. Kumar. "Nursing Care of Patients with Late-Stage Parkinson's Disease." *Journal of Neuroscience Nursing*, 35:5 (Oct. 2003): 242–251. Review.

Clifford, T. J., et al. "Burning Mouth in Parkinson's Disease Sufferers." *Gerodontology*, 15:2 (1998): 73–78.

Fukayo, S., et al. "Oral Health of Patients with Parkinson's Disease:

Factors Related to Their Better Dental Status." *Tohoku Journal of Experimental Medicine,* 201:3 (Nov. 2003): 171–179.

Kale, R., and M. Menken. "Who Should Look after People with Parkinson's Disease?" *British Medical Journal,* 328:7431 (Jan. 10, 2004): 62–63.


TREATMENT

Anderson, K. E., and J. Mullins. "Behavioral Changes Associated with Deep Brain Stimulation Surgery for Parkinson's Disease." *Current Neurology and Neuroscience Reports,* 3:4 (July 2003): 306–313. Review.

Brooks, D. J. "Safety and Tolerability of COMT Inhibitors." *Neurology,* 62 (1 Suppl. 1) (Jan. 13, 2004): S39–46. Review.

Chan, D. K. "The Art of Treating Parkinson Disease in the Older Patient." *Australian Family Physician,* 32:11 (Nov. 2003): 927–931.

Eskandar, E. N., et al. "Surgery for Parkinson Disease in the United States, 1996 to 2000: Practice Patterns, Short-Term Outcomes, and Hospital Charges in a Nationwide Sample." *Journal of Neurosurgery,* 99:5 (Nov. 2003): 863–871.

Fink, D. J., J. Glorioso, and M. Mata. "Therapeutic Gene Transfer with Herpes-Based Vectors: Studies in Parkinson's Disease and Motor Nerve Regeneration." *Experimental Neurology,* 184 (Suppl. 1) (Nov. 2003): S19–24.

Freed, C. R., et al. "Do Patients with Parkinson's Disease Benefit from Embryonic Dopamine Cell Transplantation? *Journal of Neurology,* 250 (Suppl. 3) (Oct. 2003):S44–46.

Hauser, R. A. "Levodopa/Carbidopa/Entacapone (Stalevo)." *Neurology,* 62 (1 Suppl. 1) (Jan. 13, 2004): S64–71.

Herzog, J., et al. "Two-Year Follow-up of Subthalamic Deep Brain Stimulation in Parkinson's Disease." *Movement Disorders,* 18:11 (Nov. 2003): 1332–1337.

Hurelbrink, C. B., and R. A. Barker. "The Potential of GDNF as a

Treatment for Parkinson's Disease." *Experimental Neurology,* 185:1 (Jan. 2004): 1–6.

Olanow, C. W. "Present and Future Directions in the Management of Motor Complications in Patients with Advanced PD." *Neurology,* 61 (6 Suppl. 3) (Sept. 23, 2003): S24–33. Review.

———. "The Scientific Basis for the Current Treatment of Parkinson's Disease." *Annual Review of Medicine,* 55 (2004): 41–60.

Panikar, D., and A. Kishore. "Deep Brain Stimulation for Parkinson's Disease." *Neurology India,* 51:2 (June 2003): 167–175. Review.

Park, S., et al. "Genetically Modified Human Embryonic Stem Cells Relieve Symptomatic Motor Behavior in a Rat Model of Parkinson's Disease." *Neuroscience Letters,* 353:2 (Dec. 19, 2003): 91–94.

Rascol, O., et al. "Limitations of Current Parkinson's Disease Therapy." *Annals of Neurology,* 53 (Suppl. 3) (2003): S3–12; discussion S12–15. Review.

Romrell, J., H. H. Fernandez, and M. S. Okun. "Rationale for Current Therapies in Parkinson's Disease." *Expert Opinion on Pharmacotherapy,* 4:10 (Oct. 2003): 1747–1761. Review.

## PSYCHOLOGICAL ISSUES

Askenasy, J. J. "Sleep Disturbances in Parkinsonism." *Journal of Neural Transmission,* 110:2 (Feb. 2003): 125–150. Review.

Bosboom, J. L., D. Stoffers, and E. C. Wolters. "The Role of Acetylcholine and Dopamine in Dementia and Psychosis in Parkinson's Disease." *Journal of Neural Transmission,* 65 (Suppl. 2003): 185–195. Review.

D'Souza, C., et al. "Management of Psychosis in Parkinson's Disease." *International Journal of Clinical Practice,* 57:4 (May 2003): 295–300. Review.

McDonald, W. M., I. H. Richard, and M. R. DeLong. "Prevalence, Etiology, and Treatment of Depression in Parkinson's Disease." *Biological Psychiatry,* 54:3 (Aug. 1, 2003): 363–375. Review.

Poewe, W. "Psychosis in Parkinson's Disease." *Movement Disorders,* 18 (Suppl. 6) (Sept. 2003): S80–87.

Thanvi, B. R., et al. "Neuropsychiatric Non-Motor Aspects of Parkinson's Disease." *Postgrad Medical Journal,* 79:936 (Oct. 2003):
561–565.


MISCELLANEOUS

Biousse, V., et al. "Newman Ophthalmologic Features of Parkinson's
Disease." *Neurology,* 62:2 (Jan. 27, 2004): 177–180.
Emerit, J., M. Edeas, and F. Bricaire. "Neurodegenerative Diseases
and Oxidative Stress." *Biomedical Pharmacotherapy,* 58:1 (Jan.
2004): 39–46.
Ragonese, P., et al. "A Case-Control Study on Cigarette, Alcohol, and
Coffee Consumption Preceding Parkinson's Disease."
*Neuroepidemiology,* 22:5 (Sept.–Oct. 2003): 297–304.

# Index